Ethics, Power and Policy

The Future of Nursing in the NHS

Stephen Wilmot

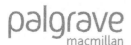

First published 2003 by
PALGRAVE MACMILLAN
Houndmills, Basingstoke, Hampshire RG21 6XS and
175 Fifth Avenue, New York, N.Y. 10010
Companies and representatives throughout the world

PALGRAVE MACMILLAN is the global academic imprint of the Palgrave Macmillan division of St. Martin's Press, LLC and of Palgrave Macmillan Ltd. Macmillan® is a registered trademark in the United States, United Kingdom and other countries. Palgrave is a registered trademark in the European Union and other countries.

ISBN 0–333–948246

This book is printed on paper suitable for recycling and made from fully managed and sustained forest sources.

A catalogue record for this book is available from the British Library.

10   9   8   7   6   5   4   3   2   1
12   11   10   09   08   07   06   05   04   03

Printed and bound in Great Britain by
J.W. Arrowsmith Ltd, Bristol.

Contents

Acknowledgements

I wish to acknowledge the help of the following in the preparation of this book.

Students and Colleagues at the University of Derby. It was through working and debating with them that the ideas behind the book germinated and developed.

Editorial staff of Palgrave Macmillan and their freelance associates. Working with them was like booking to fly economy and then discovering I had been upgraded to first class.

1 Health

Introduction

This chapter is untypical of the rest of the book in that it makes very little mention of nursing. Instead it lays the groundwork for what comes later by focusing on the concept that underpins the entire discussion – that is, the concept of health. The chapter explores some of the attempts that have been made in recent decades to achieve a workable definition of health, and also suggests a way of conceptualising health which does not require a precise definition but which nonetheless allows clear thinking about its significance. The concept of health is linked to some moral considerations, which may help to clarify that significance, and also may begin to provide a moral and political framework for health care.

What is health?

During the past fifty years there have been many attempts to define health. Ordinary citizens in many societies throughout the world have been asked for their definitions of health by academic investigators, and have offered a range of answers.

Philosophers and social scientists have attempted to bring the concept into a firm and durable framework. Influential groups, notably the medical profession, have sought to persuade the rest of the community of their view of the nature of health, with varying degrees of success. Governments and international bodies have sought a definition which allows them to frame policy and allocate resources in a rational way. As we start the twenty-first century the range of definitions is more diverse than ever before, and the prospect of consensus correspondingly less. In this chapter, I propose to explore some of the issues raised by this situation, and to consider how we can understand health care as a morally coherent enterprise in the context of these considerations.

We may pose the question as follows: is there is a universal idea called 'health' which means the same wherever we are and whoever we are with? When we try to define health are we doing something equivalent to defining (for instance) a particular kind of bacterium? In the case of the bacterium we would expect to find a class of objects (individual bacteria) existing independently of the classifier, with enough in common to allow a common label, with a common definition, to be attached to them. Is this the case with health? The answer probably is that it is not. The label of health does not seem to attach to one class of clearly identifiable phenomena. It can be connected with a number of objectively identifiable phenomena concerned with the functions of the body, but it cannot be *equated* with any of these. It can equally be connected to subjective experiences and interior states, which are very difficult to identify and measure reliably. The further we go into the question, the more difficult it becomes.

There have been many attempts to define health, and three of these are enough to provide ample illustration of the difficulties involved. The biomedical model, as described by numerous commentators over recent decades (e.g. Seedhouse 1986; Bunton *et al.* 1995) defines health as the absence of disease. It locates health firmly in the physical arena, and in the context of the physical sciences, thereby offering what appear to be clear and objective criteria for judging the degree of health of an organism. However, the problem is that the biomedical model of health is purely negative. It does not, in truth, define health at all, but is primarily concerned with disease. Health is an absence, not a presence, and if we are seeking a positive concept of health, the biomedical model does not provide this.

By contrast, the functional model of health put forward by Parsons (1972) is essentially social, using the ability to perform normal social roles as the yardstick of health. So whereas the biomedical model identifies health with the same phenomena wherever we are in the world, the functional model is uncompromisingly relativist. The kind of characteristics needed to participate in socially normal activities will vary enormously depending on the norms of the particular society. The physical and psychological characteristics enabling someone to be a member of a warrior aristocracy will be very different from those enabling someone to be a member of a peasant community, or a mercantile bourgeoisie. If this is the yardstick of health, as the functionalist would argue, then health will vary also. The problem with this definition is that the concept of health almost disappears into the concept of normality, and in terms of its practical implications it probably would disappear, if fully applied. If we want to retain the idea of health as a distinct category, functionalism is unlikely to help us.

A third definition of health is embodied in the constitution of the World Health Organization (WHO 1946), which equates health with complete physical, mental and social well-being. A close link between health and well-being appeals to common sense, but an agreed and consistent definition of well-being is impossible to attain, and on that basis the definition fails. Seedhouse (1986) points out that the content of the experience of well-being will vary in accordance with culture and personality. As to the degree of well-being, how much is enough? The WHO refers to complete well-being, which suggests a state of perfection. Clearly this is unattainable in ordinary living. For these reasons it is doubtful whether it can offer a reliable or objective yardstick for health.

It is clear that the three models of health discussed above work from very different bases, and operate in very different conceptual paradigms. This makes it very difficult to compare them. And it should be remembered that they are simply three of the better-known definitions of health. There are many more. The problem that emerges here is not that we are unable to arrive at a definition of health. On the contrary, the problem is that we can arrive at too many definitions, and that they cannot be reconciled. The difficulties with the three definitions I have touched on so far are repeated elsewhere. Writing in a nursing context, McBean (1997) identifies eight definitions of health, mostly drawn from other writers on nursing. Looking at the proliferation of such definitions in nursing literature, she finds no less than five in one nursing text (Marriner-Tomey 1989). The process also shows itself in the business of measuring health. Bowling's (1998) discussion of measuring health is very useful in overviewing a range of instruments for different assessment foci, but it also highlights the bewildering diversity of underpinning conceptual frameworks, many of which could reasonably claim to offer a definition of health. Anderson *et al.*'s (1993: p. 373) comment on this issue – ' a positive conception of health is difficult to measure because of the lack of agreement over its definition' – seems entirely apposite here. It is fair to say that these uncertainties are also reflected in lay definitions of health. Blaxter's (1987) classic study of health perceptions in the population produced a considerable variety of perceptions, which provided little in the way of a bedrock for a shared definition.

Coping with multiple definitions of health

This abundance of definitions of health has given rise to three kinds of response. One of these is to seek to redefine heath in a way that is more rigorous and workable than has been achieved so far, using the experience of decades of struggle with the concept in order to learn from past mistakes. This is the approach taken by Seedhouse (1986), who has developed a model of health as the foundations of achievement; that which allows people to achieve their chosen and biological potential. This definition has affinities with all of the three definitions I discussed above, but its practical implications are likely to appeal most to those otherwise inclined toward the WHO definition. Seedhouses's project is to provide a definition which is not just philosophically coherent but also practically workable. The danger with this approach is that, whatever the quality of the definition, it will simply be placed alongside its competitors in an undifferentiated field. To some degree this seems to have happened in this case.

The second response is to accept elusiveness and uncertainty as in some way essential to the nature of health. This is the approach taken by Gadamer (1996), who sees health as invisible, or (using different imagery) weightless. He comes nearest to a definition by using the concept of health as equilibrium, but it is the weightless sensation created by that equilibrium that emerges most strongly from his discussion. Fox (1999), taking an explicitly postmodern view of health, develops a concept he calls 'arche-health' which is health as choice, transformation and openness, as opposed to health as a fixed entity or idea. The two approaches are very different in their conceptualisation of health, but show a similar strategy and style in dealing with the problem of defining health.

The third response is to approach health as a social construct; not to seek any essential meaning in the concept but simply to understand its behaviour in the contexts in which it can be identified. Health is a concept of importance in most, if not all societies and cultures, and its manifestations and variations between cultures and subcultures have been closely studied by writers such as Helman (1994). Health is also a concept of political importance in contemporary western society and particular definitions of health are the focus of various political agendas. For instance O'Brien (1995) provides an interesting account of the politics discernible behind contemporary public health, recruiting for its purposes the WHO definition of health.

I do not propose to pursue further the question of whether there is a 'true' definition of health among the plethora of competing versions. Seedhouse, Gadamer and Fox would, I suspect, not be happy with the idea of a 'true' definition in any case, and it could be argued that they are seeking workable perspectives for their different agendas, rather than 'true' ones. It may be that for many purposes health can best be understood as a social construct, and that its meaning is context-dependent. However, this does not remove health from the political or moral agenda. Other important phenomena can be understood as socially constructed, but that does not mean that they are not a proper object of debate and deliberation, or a proper focus of public policy. We may take poverty as an example. Poverty is constructed in different ways in different societies, and someone who is poor in one society may not be so in another. Poverty does not exist independently of social definitions. But that does not diminish its importance, for individuals and societies. The same goes for health. But what we *can* infer from the proposition that health is a social construct is that we may not be able to arrive at a stable and satisfactory definition of it, because it cannot be observed 'out there' as a measurable phenomenon.

Health as a good

Instead of attempting to add yet another definition of health to the existing list I propose take a rather different approach. I shall briefly explore health by considering the way we apply the concept, and by relating that to other concepts with which it is sometimes associated. Interesting linkages of socially valued ideas can often be found embedded in ordinary language, and this is certainly true of health. We can find it in the 'health, wealth and happiness' triad beloved of English wedding guests proposing toasts to the happy couple. In the folk wisdom of proverbs, health is associated with wisdom ('healthy, wealthy and wise'), while in the modern context of western popular culture we frequently associate health with beauty. So it is useful to consider whether these associations reflect some real commonality; whether health, wealth, happiness, wisdom and beauty have anything of substance in common that deepens our understanding of health.

Despite their differences, I would argue that happiness, wisdom, beauty and health do have a crucial similarity in the way we apply them, in that they are all terms which are used to combine evaluative and descriptive elements. With all of them it is possible to identify criteria in an object or person qualifying them as happy, wise, beautiful or healthy. In every case those criteria are the subject of disagreement, but those disagreements are in themselves indications that the participants believe that such criteria are possible to arrive at. However, to call a person happy or wise or beautiful is not simply to describe them. It is also to evaluate them or their situation or actions. Likewise to refer to anything or anyone as 'healthy' is almost certainly to commend them as well as describe them. We can contrast this with words such as 'red', which are purely descriptive, and the word 'good', which is often used in a way that is purely evaluative, with no descriptive content. Happiness, wisdom, beauty and health all carry within their meaning the positive valuation of 'good' but also offer a description of that to which they are being applied.

The idea of wealth, associated in sayings and proverbs with health, happiness and wisdom, provides an interesting contrast. I would suggest that wealth is fundamentally different from the other four concepts and that what divides health, happiness, beauty and wisdom from wealth is that the former are seen as goods in themselves, while the latter is seen as a means to a range of desirable outcomes – the things that money can buy. This is not an absolute divide, because wisdom and health can also be seen as means to other things – particularly happiness. But they do not depend on this. Health and wisdom are also desirable in themselves in a way that wealth is not. Wealth is not an evaluative term in the sense that the others are. Although we know that it is valued in western culture and many other cultures as a general character-istic, and we may value it ourselves, that is a contingent fact dependent on context. By contrast, the other list, including health, are significantly more free of context.

But what is it about wisdom, beauty, happiness and health that make them valued? The answer is probably different in every case. Mill (1962) argued that it is in our nature to value happiness, implying a fundamental law of psychology. Modern psychology sees the matter in more complex terms, but it still makes reason-able sense to say that we value what we enjoy, and that happiness is by its nature enjoyable. It is also true to say that in most cases we have no difficulty recognising when we are happy and when we are unhappy. By contrast our ability to appreciate beauty and wisdom can be argued to depend on a degree of cultivated sensibility, which will be aesthetic in the case of beauty and intellectual in the case of wisdom. To some degree we need to learn to recognise and value these goods.

In the case of health the question arises as to whether our ability to value health also depends on a learned sensibility equivalent to the moral and the aesthetic, or whether we find it immediately and intuitively attractive. We certainly dislike the absence of health as we dislike the absence of happiness. Nobody enjoys being ill. But the appreciation of positive health may require an inner tuning and awareness that needs cultivation. Perhaps we need to become 'health-conscious' to appreciate positive health, as we need to be morally and aesthetically aware to appreciate justice and beauty. Gadamer (1996) suggests that health is very difficult to experience directly, maybe even impossible. Perhaps if we create a continuum with beauty and wisdom at one end and happiness at the other, we can place health in between, representing an inter-mediate zone between the spontaneous and innate appreciation of happiness, and the learned appreciation of beauty and wisdom.

So far we have compared health with wisdom, happiness and beauty. But we can understand more of what is valuable about health if we introduce another valued concept into the discussion. Justice, like health and the others, combines descriptive and evalu-ative meaning. There are criteria for a just act or a just decision, the presence of which can be verified, and to characterise an act as just is partly to say that it meets these criteria. However to say a decision is just is also to commend it. Justice may lead to other good outcomes, but irrespective of this it is seen as good in itself. In these respects it resembles health, beauty, wisdom, and happiness.

However, the kind of commendation involved in ascribing justice is different from that involved with the other concepts discussed. This is because justice is a moral good. We value it because it is intrinsically right to value it. We *ought* to value it. In the case of happiness it makes more sense to say that we value it because it is in our nature to do so. Happiness always attracts us because of what we are. Justice only attracts us if we understand why we ought to value it. It appeals to our moral sense of right and wrong rather than to our natural desires. Our ability to appreciate justice represents a higher sensibility that requires learning and cultivation, and in that sense it resembles beauty and wisdom. However, the sensibility required in the case of justice is a moral sensibility, not an aesthetic or intellectual sensibility. In the same way, health differs from justice in that, though we may need a degree of developed sensibility to fully appreciate health, that is not a moral sensibility, and health is not a moral good.

So far I have suggested that we can see health as a good whose value is not confined to a specific culture or cultures. I have suggested that it is not a moral good, like justice, but occupies a different category alongside beauty, wisdom and happiness. None of these are moral goods as such. But it is worth adding here that at least two of them have been used by moral philosophers to provide a basis for moral judgements. Happiness has been used by the Utilitarians to provide a practical basis for moral goodness. The utilitarian attempt to ground morality in happiness is expressed in Mill's (1962) dictum that an act is good insofar as it tends to maximise happiness. The logic of choosing happiness was that it is universally sought and valued, as is no other good. We could also argue that Kant based his system of ethics on wisdom (Paton 1978). In fact he always referred to reason rather than wisdom, but his principle – that right actions can only be identified through the use of reason to see our duty – implies something indistinguishable from many definitions of wisdom. If these goods relate so closely to morality, we might expect that health, with so many characteristics in common, will do likewise. The next section explores this relationship.

Health and morality

The relationship between health and morality is complex. Moral arguments have been used widely to support the promotion of health and provision of health care. Such arguments will in fact form a significant theme of the rest of this book. They have taken various forms, and have given different statuses to health. Writers such as Beauchamp and Childress (1994) have linked health to general well-being (as with the WHO) arguing that we can base moral judgements on a broad basis of well-being, and that this can include health. This gives health an important status as a basis of morality, and argues that all actions that promote health or effective health care are morally right actions (and that those with the opposite effect are wrong). However, the difficulty of recruiting health to this purpose is the very one that we have been considering. Happiness, the original utilitarian yardstick, is an experience that everyone can recognise for themselves and in a sense needs no defining, although early utilitarians such as Bentham (1962) tried very hard to define and quantify it. Health is less immediately recognisable, and there is not enough consensus on its definition for it to provide a secure basis for morality. However, this does not apply to all aspects of health. I said earlier that ill-health is recognisable to most of us even though positive health is neither immediately recognisable nor a matter of consensus. If we use happiness or well-being as a utilitarian basis for moral judgements, then we can argue that ill-health reduces well-being and happiness, and that anything that reduces ill-health will therefore promote well-being and happiness. So if we confine ourselves to the prevention and treatment of ill-health the utilitarian basis for justifying health promotion and health care as moral goals is stronger.

Some ethical systems, for instance those of Kant and the Existentialists, place particular emphasis on autonomy and the making of choices, rather than on happiness or well-being. The moral value of health and health care must then rest on the importance of health for autonomy. This is part of the basis of Doyal and Gough's (1991) need-based argument. They see social participation as a fundamental need, and life and autonomy as the necessary underpinnings of this. Ill-health clearly impairs autonomy in various ways, and provision to prevent or treat ill-health is thereby justified. A related argument proposes that because health is an underpinning of individual liberty, at least some of the same rights that we might ascribe to an individual in relation to their liberty might be ascribable in relation to their health. The key rights here would be what are sometimes termed 'negative rights', that is rights not to be interfered with. The right not to have one's liberty impaired or limited place a duty on others simply to leave the individual alone. A similar argument can be applied to health in that we might claim a right to be left alone to enjoy our health, and not to have it impaired or damaged. However, though this might justify the prevention of pollution and other damaging activities, it does not entail a right to health care as such. And this brings us to the crucial connection between health and health care.

Health and health care

I have argued that health can be linked to moral good in a number of ways. Some of these linkages support the notion that efforts to prevent or cure ill-health are morally right. This gives a particular significance and status to health care. But health care has come to signify a wide range of activities that go beyond the more limited meaning of 'care'. It includes advice, investigation, treatment, monitoring, screening and health promotion. The bulk of these activities are focused on responding to illness, and they reflect the dominance of the biomedical model of health within the health care system. The importance of the value of health in underpinning health care, and the close link to moral good, can be seen from a consideration of groups mainly involved in providing health care. Typically in the western world, health care, like other socially valued activities, has been made the territory of professional groups. Nursing and Medicine draw heavily on the idea of vocation as a motivation for engaging in their activities, and have professional codes which are strongly ethically oriented. Looking around the world, it is unusual for health care to be a purely commercial activity. The United States comes closest among the developed countries, and in reality its system is some way from being purely commercial. Generally, health care has been seen as an activity with a strong non-material element to the motivation of its workers. This would suggest that health care is truly a moral project.

However, the commitment of these key professional groups to the non-commercial activity of caring is not the whole story, and other factors, such as power, come into the health care picture. Nurses and doctors both enjoy significant degrees of social prestige though they manifest in very different ways, generally to the advantage of the doctors. Traditionally the medical profession has been associated with the more interventive activity of treatment, and the nursing profession with the less interventive activity of care (in the narrow sense), and this association has been to the doctors' advantage in terms of social power. The patient's role has tended to be one of passivity, as the origin of the word 'patient' would suggest, and there is plenty of evidence that patients have real difficulty maintaining a sense of initiative and control, particularly in the face of medical power and prestige (Nettleton 1995). If health is an underpinning of autonomy, and this is part of the basis of a claim to health care, it could be argued that those seeking to restore health are justified in this by the restoration of autonomy. But the fact that much health care seems to have the opposite effect, in disempowering the patient, suggests that there are other agendas at work. Some commentators, notably Illich (1995), have argued that the doctor-dominated biomedical version of health care is in fact an instrument of oppression, and does more harm than good to people's health, not least because it disempowers them in a particularly comprehensive way. There is evidence that patients are not in truth quite so dominated by their doctors as the radical view supposes (Nettleton 1995), but it is nonetheless clearly an unequal relationship.

So it is one thing to say that health is a good and ought to be promoted, but it is quite another to say that the dominant model of health and health care offers the best way of promoting health. If the process of promoting that good also does unacceptable harm, we should look for different ways of achieving our goal. Indeed, there are alternative models of health care. Public health and health promotion, particularly in the framework of what has come to be known as 'the New Public Health' represents such an alternative approach, involving the positive promotion of health and the goal of empowerment of the population. However, commentators such as O'Brien (1995) argue that a power agenda is present here also. Its efficacy in reducing health inequalities has also been questioned (Foster 1996). So a major problem arises for those seeking to provide health care as part of a moral agenda, in that the activity seems indelibly contaminated by the dishonest and manipulative use of professional and state power.

However, the moral significance of health care does not lie simply in its efficacy. If it is morally commendable for its outcome, it is commendable for other reasons also. Its commendability also lies in the nature of the relationship being expressed in the activity of care. At a one-to-one level the valuation of the other person and the giving of self involved in caring activities carries with it a moral significance that goes beyond the effectiveness of health care in improving health (Noddings 1986). And on a collective level, the provision of care expresses inclusion and social solidarity, providing an important acknowledgement of citizenship. It is clear that much health care does not in fact improve health, certainly not in the biomedical sense. In the case of patients with chronic or terminal diseases, such care may improve health in the WHO sense of improving well-being, but that is more difficult to measure objectively.

The commendability of health care does not rest entirely on its ability to restore or promote health because it has never, and never will, succeed in doing this in all cases where care is appropriate.

The state and health care

Later in the book we shall be considering the role of the individual in attending to their own health, and the role of the state in organising the provision of health care. However, at this stage we need to begin to consider the difficulties that have arisen over the issue of the state's role. For most of the first half of the twentieth century the belief that the state ought to take the lead in organising health care steadily gained ground, and in the UK the argument for state involvement seemed to triumph in 1948 with the foundation of the National Health Service. In the rest of Europe patterns of state involvement varied with political complexions, but the state took a leading role in most countries. In the UK the state set up and ran a health service financed out of taxation. Some of the impetus for this development came from political calculation, but as Klein (1995) acknowledges, it was also

underpinned by essentially moral perspectives on health, in particular views of health as a public good and as an individual right.
Health care was one of a small number of provisions to be organised in this way, which reflected the social valuation placed upon
health.

The dominant model of health for most of the twentieth
century was the biomedical model, and the National Health Service reflected that model, being in truth a service to treat the
sick. However, in the final decades of the century several things
happened to change this situation. Among these were major
cultural developments, which led to changes in attitudes to health
(described by writers such as Bordo 1993) and also changes in
attitudes to public services (see, for instance, Francome and Marks
1996). Increased diversity, individualisation and consumerisation
of the culture led to a more complex view of health among both
the public and the professionals. This change included greater
emphasis on health promotion, the increasing inclusion of well-
being into health, the introduction of ideas from complementary
therapies, the commodification of health-related experiences
(such as diet and fitness regimes) as leisure and life-style options,
and an increased preoccupation with risk (Bunton and Burrows
1995). Many of these changes, particularly in relation to consumerisation, led to diminishing tolerance of a public service
which provided a relatively undifferentiated product, insensitive
to individual preferences. At the same time the NHS became
increasingly expensive, as treatments developed and the population aged.

Since the mid-1980s successive governments have struggled to
respond to these changes. In particular they have tried to achieve a
new consensus on the issue of who should provide what in relation
to health and health care and to what standard. This has involved
reviewing several boundaries. The aspects of health that are the
business of the NHS have been extended to include individual
lifestyles (by the pre-1997 Conservative government) and health
inequalities (by the post-1997 Labour government), though it is
not clear that an effective way has been found to achieve real
changes in either of these areas. At the same time the NHS
struggles to sustain a basic undifferentiated service, and is constantly vulnerable to sudden changes in demand. This has led to
some public discontent. As the use of private health insurance has

increased, there has been doubt as to the willingness of the taxpayer to finance the improvements necessary to enable the NHS to meet users expectations.

The difficulty in finding a consensus on what is required and what should be expected is not peculiar to health. Changes in British society since the 1940s have meant that the belief in a common culture and set of values which was part of the national self-image (though not entirely accurate) has receded a good deal, and a more relativist perspective is widespread (Giddens 1991). To return for a moment to the goods I compared with health – beauty, happiness, and wisdom – the general view on all of these is likely to be more diverse than it was fifty years ago, with a wider belief that there is no single formula for any of these goods. The other crucial development relevant to these goods is the diminution of deference to rank and expertise. People are less willing to be told by professionals or politicians what it is to be healthy, or happy, or wise, or how they might become so. In this context, the health care system needs to be able to reflect and respond to the greater complexity and volatility of the society it serves. To some degree it needs to reflect that society within itself. At the same time it needs sufficient focus and directionality to anticipate developments, to lead and to educate. It needs a mandate which allows it to do these things in a way that retains its legitimacy. It is crucial that the key personnel involved in the NHS are effective in enabling these conditions to be met.

Conclusion

The problem of achieving an agreed definition of health presents a challenge to everyone involved in health care, but I have suggested that there is a way of dealing with the concept of health that does not require a firm agreed definition but involves instead recognition of the dual nature of health as both descriptive and evaluative. Though it is not in itself a moral good, health has a very close relationship to particular moral goods, and it is these links that provide the moral and political framework for the provision of health care. In an increasingly diverse society, however, we cannot rely on a consensus on health or on health care, to guide us toward an appropriate health care system.

The rest of the book

The rest of this book is concerned with the issues considered in this chapter. It is concerned specifically with the principles upon which the health care system might base itself, if it is to be effective in responding to health care needs in contemporary society. However, it is concerned also with another dimension, which has not been a major focus of the discussion so far, but which will dominate the rest of the book. That is the role of the nursing profession in enabling the developing health care system to achieve the relevance, flexibility and legitimacy that it needs in order to be effective. Nurses, as the largest of the professional groups in the health care system, have an incalculable impact at every level on the way it operates at present. For as long as nursing exists on its present scale and in anything like its present role it will have a pivotal position in the development of health care. Its potential exceeds what has been achieved by a considerable margin. Despite appearances so far, this is a book that is primarily about nursing, and the way nursing relates to the issues discussed. The role of nursing in helping to define health and in developing health care is considered in Chapter 2, and in later chapters its relationship with the state, the patient/citizen, the organisations involved in health care, and other professions involved in health care, will be discussed in turn. Once these relationships have been explored, I shall suggest a moral and social framework for the health care system and a role for nursing within that framework. The last part of the book will explore specific issues within this overall health care scene, and consider how the role of nursing might operate in that particular context.

2 Nursing

Introduction

This chapter explores the position of the nursing profession in the health care system, historically and in the present. The values and knowledge base of the profession are considered, together with its strengths, needs and potential as a force to shape the development of health care. The discussion also acknowledges the power of medicine in health care and takes account of the relationship between the two professions.

Nurses and doctors, past and present

Nurses constitute the largest professional group involved in health care. We might expect that this kind of numerical predominance, combined with its key role in the health care process, would guarantee to nursing a position of high prestige and power in the health care system. That would be the logic of the situation. But reality is quite different. To understand the real position of nursing in the health care system it is necessary to understand one salient, overwhelming fact of history; that is, the dominance of the medical profession, and the impact of this on the position of nurses. In the relevant historical period (roughly the 500 years since the Renaissance) both doctoring and nursing in Europe have been carried out in diverse ways by diverse people. Doctoring as a paid activity was done variously by barber-surgeons, apothecaries and physicians. Nursing as a paid or recompensed activity was done by women of various social statuses, ranging from nuns to local wise-women. But during that time medicine had two major advantages over nursing in gaining dominance. First, proto-doctors had various forms of organisation, based originally on the medieval guild but developing slowly into more modern forms. Nurses had nothing to match these organisations. Second, doctors were men, and nurses were women. Gender has been a crucial factor in moulding the social relationship between the two groups during the modern period. The inequality of power between men and women in western society inevitably reflected itself in this particular relationship.

However, this does not mean that medical dominance over nursing was natural or inevitable. On the contrary it was the result of conscious strategies by the protagonists. It has been argued by Ehrenreich and English (1973) that women healers and carers presented real competition to doctors in early modern times, and that the drive on the part of doctors toward primacy in health care was in part an attempt to control this competition. If we take the period when the modern medical and nursing professions took a firm institutional shape, in the years following the mid-nineteenth century, we can identify political processes in which the medical profession gained power over key aspects of health care through skilled lobbying, negotiation and pressure. Blane (1997) describes some of the strategies used by the medical profession to gain a monopoly position in relation to health care. This process was at its height between the mid-nineteenth century and the early twentieth century. Ehrenreich and English argue that the creation of the modern nursing profession by Nightingale and her associates represents the final defeat of the woman healer as a rival to the doctor, and the 'domestication' of the nurse. Wicks (1998) suggests that this argument is overstated, but it seems true that the founders of modern nursing on the whole saw medicine as having legitimate primacy in health care, and envisaged the nurse's role as existing within the constraints imposed by that primacy. This does not mean that they saw nursing as an ancillary or supplementary activity. Nightingale was clear that nursing had a defined and distinctive role quite separate from that of medicine, and should have a management structure and organisation that expressed that separateness. But she did not see nursing as an actual or potential competitor to medicine.

It is hardly surprising, given the nineteenth century historical context, that the doctors, a group of middle-class men, showed themselves more able to gain power and influence than did the nurses, a group of middle-class and working-class women. In the mid-to-late nineteenth century the general disparity of social power between men and women within the bourgeoisie was as great as it has been in modern times. Middle-class married women were normally allowed a significant role only in the privacy of family life. Outside the confines of the home they could only expect passivity and marginality, while single women were generally marginalised within as well as outside of the home. In that social context it is remarkable that nursing managed to establish itself at all. It was a considerable achievement for a group of women to establish and legitimise a viable occupational identity in those conditions.

My brief historical introduction has emphasised gender as the crucial factor in explaining the dominance of medicine in health care. Other factors are also important. The nature of the profession as an institution has played a part in the nursing-medicine relationship. We can see professions as institutions for the organisational and ethical regulation of important and valued activities, as Parsons (1939) did. We can also see them as part of a system of social and economic control in a hierarchical economic and social system, as commentators such as Freidson (1970) have. If we take the period of the medical profession's greatest success in extending its dominance in health care, a period of ninety years from the Medical Act to the creation of the NHS, we can place these events in the context of a hierarchical society in which powerful professional groups operated as part of a system of social dominance, exerting cultural as well as economic and legal power. Nurses were unable to develop the necessary social power during that period to enjoy the full advantages of professional status, despite a number of features that qualify them as a profession. They remained lower than medicine in the class structure, and experienced subordination in the clinical setting. Medicine by contrast gained monopoly economic power by virtue of its domination of health care, and its position in terms of class and status was one of considerable advantage.

The culmination of this crucial ninety years, the creation of the National Health Service, seemed to further institutionalise medical dominance. The National Health Service as it came into being in 1948 accommodated doctors' concerns, rather than those of nurses. The nursing input into the negotiations that produced the final plan of the NHS was very limited, and both Rafferty (1992) and White (1985) show that nurses' views continued to be systematically ignored and dismissed in the early years of the NHS.

However, change is inevitable, though its form is unpredictable. Often culture and perceptions change more quickly than structures, and this is the case with nursing. From the 1960s onward nurses' perception of their own role started slowly to shift. Nurses in the UK started to feel the influence of ideas coming from nurses in the US and Australia. The US influence was particularly significant in terms of the development of nursing theory, and the building up of a distinctive knowledge base for the profession, which Meleis (1997) in the US context dates from the 1950s. The emergence of nurse advocacy offered a professional activity which in Kuhse's (1997) view allowed not only an autonomous role in relation to medicine, but also an oppositional role. During the 1980s the shift in knowledge base and professional self-concept expressed itself in the move toward a new kind of training at a higher educational and theoretical level. All these developments significantly affected nurses' perceptions of themselves.

However, the perceptions of others, and the relationships arising from this, have not necessarily changed in the same way; nor have structures. There is ample evidence of a continued assumption of dominance on the part of the medical profession in relation to nurses, and behaviour in accordance with this assumption. MacKay's (1993) hospital based study, and Williams' (2000) more recent study of primary care show that doctors still expect to dominate, seek to dominate, and to a significant degree do dominate. At the same time both studies, alongside many other similar investigations, show that that dominance is constantly challenged, usually covertly but often effectively, by nurses who have developed a range of skills and strategies to contain and circumvent medical power. Despite this, Williams expresses some pessimism about the prospect of a change in the balance of power in the crucial primary care sector. We might simplify the picture by suggesting that in interactional terms nurses resist medical dominance (see, for instance, Svensson 1996) but in social-structural terms that dominance continues to be reinforced. We might add that gender continues to be a crucial factor in the relationship. Although medicine is becoming feminised in numerical terms, it remains culturally masculine. Conversely, while the small minority of male nurse are over-represented at managerial level, they do not seem to greatly affect the gendered nature of the doctor-nurse confrontation at ground level.

These processes have taken place in structural and cultural contexts that are themselves changing. Since the 1970s government has attempted to make the NHS more rational and responsive in its working, and the resultant changes have created pressures for both medicine and nursing. Davies (1995) suggests that for most of this period nurses were virtually invisible to the planners involved in these changes, whereas doctors were seen as central to their concerns. This is probably less true of changes that have happened since 1997, but her claim seems highly credible for the period between 1974 and 1997. It has been widely supposed that the first change to significantly impact on medical power was the introduction of the internal market in 1990, and that the hospital consultants were the losers in this. If this is true, a number of commentators (for instance Dent 1995) argue that the erosion was modest. The same changes certainly put pressure on nurses in terms of working conditions. The changes of 1997 onward explicitly gave a higher profile to nurses, both in the structural arrangements for primary care, and also in the policy priorities for health promotion. But in the context of primary care they also institutionalised the power of GPs at the organisational level. So to some degree changes may have cancelled one another out, though in primary care it is too early to be certain of this.

However, the position of the medical profession has been eroded in other ways. Its social prestige in society as a whole is reduced, not because of a loss of public confidence (which remains comparatively high in both professions) but simply because medical prestige depended a good deal on a culture of deference, which is fading fast as the general public become less willing to give respect and compliance on the basis of status. At the same time it is clear that the biomedical model of healthcare, which has also dominated, along with the doctors, for most of the past fifty years, is now in retreat. The shift to a broader view of health, and to a focus on health promotion and public health has been progressing since the 1970s in the thinking of many organisations, and since the late 1980s in government thinking, exemplified in documents such as *The Health of the Nation* (Department of Health 1992).

Nursing – fitness for purpose

My argument in the rest of this book is that health care in the UK will have to change the basis of its legitimacy if it is to be effective, and part of that change will inevitably affect the positions of the medical profession and the nursing profession. This argument is developed further in Chapters 3 and 7, but I need to begin it here for the sake of the present discussion. My central point is that the status of medical science and the medical profession has provided the foundation for public acceptance of the operation of the NHS for fifty years, but that the basis of that legitimacy is disappearing, and the legitimacy of medicine will be threatened also. I will argue, in addition, that nursing has a crucial role in responding to this situation. Partly this will depend on nursing being able to deploy equivalent skills to those deployed by the medical profession in the late nineteenth century, in exerting influence. Those skills will be discussed in a later chapter, but it is important initially to consider the assets that the profession brings to the situation. I shall begin this by considering the values, ethics and knowledge base of nursing.

Value base and knowledge base are both problematic concepts because they assume that a set of ideas or beliefs are held in common in a homogenous way within a professional group, and this is clearly not true. Individual knowledge and beliefs vary within any such group. However, two factors make it worthwhile to consider these questions. One is that we know that certain professional groups do have some shared ideas in specific areas, which make them on average more similar to their fellow professionals than they are to people from outside their profession. The other is that the nursing profession is not simply a collection of individuals, but is also an institution with a structure of formal and informal components, centring historically on the United Kingdom Central Council (UKCC), and now on the Nursing and Midwifery Council (NMC), which can in some senses speak to the outside world for, and even as, the profession. So the value-base of nursing can be assessed from a number of sources representing these aspects of the profession. Its code of conduct is based on a set of values identified explicitly or implicitly by the UKCC (1992) and the NMC (2002), while its canon of writing on nursing ethics, and on related topics represents the more explicit elements in the shared body of knowledge. By contrast the views and actions of nurses represent the non-institutional dimension of professional values, the beliefs of individual practitioners.

There are clearly epistemological problems about all these sources of evidence. We might ask whether a code of conduct can be seen as representing anything, given that it may not represent the values of any one individual. It is indeed very likely that a code of conduct will be the result of a process of negotiation, the outcomes of which represents the beliefs of no one person. How will this then relate to the real morality of nurses? Pattison (2001) argues strongly that codes in general, and the UKCC code in particular, fail signally to provide a workable ethical framework, partly because they fail to accord with the moral insights that nurses gain from life and professional experience. If so the code is a flawed source of information. Likewise expression of values in the literature represents in each case the perceptions of the writer, and we cannot be sure that they represent anyone else at all, or that they have any direct or indirect impact on the actions of nurses. Our third source of evidence, the actions of individual nurses may also not accurately express their values. It is clear that nurses feel conflicting pressures on them and that their desire to act in accordance with their professional values is often counterbalanced by pressures from colleagues, employers or patients to act otherwise. This leaves the fourth source of evidence, the expressed views and beliefs of individual nurses. These may in many respects be the 'purest' expression of nursing values but they may also be the most evanescent and insubstantial.

On the basis of the above problems we may be tempted to abandon any attempt to understand nursing values. However, because the concept of nursing values is a composite one rather than a unitary one, and must be discovered through a range of different kinds of evidence, this does not render the concept meaningless. What we find is that the evidence from these diverse sources is reasonably consistent and a similar profile emerges from each source considered. We find that a distinctive if problematic set of core values can be identified. First, nursing values tend to be individualist rather than collectivist. We can see this from the emphasis among nurses on the care of the individual patient, and their commitment to the patient's health, well-being, dignity and autonomy (Kuhse *et al.* 1997; Robertson 1996). We can also find a strong emphasis on duty as an individual commitment, incumbent on the nurse and sometimes incumbent on others also. For instance Dalley (1993) found that nurses were more comfortable with the idea of a caring duty on the part of relatives than were, for instance, social workers. The nursing code of professional conduct reflects a similar set of values, with a strong focus on the dignity and well-being of the individual patient. The code is to some degree balanced between consequentialist and deontological ethical orientations, with the deontological pre-dominating somewhat. The unique value of the individual is iden-tified in a number of clauses in the code, and the nurse's specific duty to that individual is also strongly expressed. Though some of the clauses express an essentially utilitarian perspective, seeking to maximise well-being, this is the weaker of the two themes. The strong individualism of nursing values comes through again in this context.

Writers on nursing values variously identify care (Benner and Wrubel 1989), well-being, health (Cusveller 1998) respect for rights, respect for life, and the dignity of the individual (Fagermoen 1997) as central to nursing. Seedhouse (2000) identifies the central purpose of nursing, and therefore its prime value-focus, as working for health. This is echoed from empirical evidence by Smith *et al.* (1999) who found some evidence of a generational shift among nurses toward the idea of promoting health as the main profes-sional goal. Some writers also identify an expectation upon the nurse, which goes beyond the idea of explicit and limited profes-sional duties into an area of moral excellence and self-sacrifice. Edwards (1996) refers to this as the supererogatory nurse. Though he questions whether such expectations make any ethical or profes-sional sense, their power is undeniable.

The canon of ethics literature in nursing provides an interesting background to the other evidence on nursing values. Generally discussion of nursing ethics in standard texts tends to focus round two perspectives, the deontological and the consequentialist. The deontological – duty-based – perspective is best exemplified in the moral philosophy of Immanuel Kant, with its focus on the primacy of duty and the fundamental significance of respect for persons (Paton 1978). Consequentialism, the principle of judging the rightness of an action by its consequences rather than by its nature or intentions, is best exemplified by utilitarianism, the philosophy of John Stuart Mill (1962) who saw the maximisation of happiness as the most rational and appropriate yardstick for moral good. These perspectives provide two of the theoretical cornerstones of nursing ethics as they do in the wider body of literature concerned with health care ethics. They create a theme that tends to express itself throughout nursing ethics and health care ethics, the balancing of two very different, but equally rational and humane philosophies. Texts do not on the whole advocate one perspective against the other, and the consensus favours a synthesis in principle even though such a synthesis would be at risk of being incoherent, given the very different premises of the two philosophies. Another solution that is not exactly a synthesis but combines the two perspectives at a lower level of abstraction is the use of the four-principle system popularised by Beauchamp and Childress (1994), the four principles being Beneficence, Non-Malificence, Justice and Autonomy. Edwards (1996) has strongly advocated and exemplified the use of this system in nursing ethics.

However, there is another dimension to the nursing ethics canon that reflects a more distinctive nursing flavour, and that is the principle of care, involving a position of personal commitment and empathy toward the patient. It is a principle advocated by a number of writers, and is seen as reflecting a specifically nursing viewpoint. Van Hooft (1999) sees it as a virtue. Benner and Wrubel (1989) present it as an antidote to technicalised nursing, and draw a good deal on existentialism (particularly Heidegger) for philosophical underpinning of the concept. It has also been identified as an appropriate ethical principle for a predominantly female profession, in that it reflects a female approach to ethics. In this, ideas from Gilligan (1982) and Noddings (1986) are influential. However, care has also been criticised as representing a practical principle disguised as a moral principle. Allmark (1995) and Kuhse (1997) both argue that care is not intrinsically morally right, unless it is undertaken for the right reasons. This issue is partly reducible to the question of what is an ethical principle and what is not, and the answer to this depends on the theory of meta-ethics we use. It also resolves round our precise definition of care, and the kind of care that we are applying. As Edwards (2001) points out, writing in an existentialist framework, different levels of care have very different implications in relation to human agency.

Ethical issues in nursing reflect some of the tensions generated by nursing values. The issue of conscientious objection has been an important one in nursing. The function of the individual conscience in motivating the nurse connects back to the idea of the supererogatory nurse, but the strong moral motivation of the nurse may lead into difficulties in such areas as abortion and euthanasia, where the paradox of a strong caring commitment blocking a nurse from her professional duty has raised a certain amount of controversy. The individualism of nursing values is also placed in the spotlight in situations of industrial dispute, where the collective interests of nurses, (and sometimes the collective interests of patients also) have come into conflict with the nurse's individual duty to individual patients, a problem identified inter alia by Tschudin and Hunt (1997). Both of these situations represent a conflict between moral priorities, between rights, and to some degree between duties.

Nursing knowledge is closely connected with nursing values, and reflects some of the same features. It is a cumulative, composite phenomenon, identifiable at several different levels, and the complexity that the body of nursing knowledge has developed over the decades can be readily seen from work such as that of Nicoll (1997). Nursing knowledge is embodied first in the actions of nurses, and the knowledge that informs those actions. It is also located in the requirements and activities of nurse education, and can be seen as emerging from the tension between the national bodies that oversee nurse education, and the institutions and personnel that actually provide it. It is pointless trying to establish which of these levels should have priority in the definition, as all are equally significant. Nursing like many other professions struggles with a theory-practice gap. Nursing writers have identified a range of different levels of abstraction in nursing theory, and the more abstract meta-level of nursing theorising is at a considerable distance from the concreteness of much nursing practice. Because nursing knowledge seeks to accommodate such a range of different levels and domains, it is open to the criticism of being over-inclusive and incoherent. This is a point made by Seedhouse (2000), who argues that the 'integrative tendency' in nursing culture has led to uncritical over-inclusiveness of ideas and lack of rigour in thinking.

In practice, however, the focus of nursing is individual patient care, and nurses have as a group and individually accumulated a great deal of knowledge and skill in this area. Recent evidence suggests that nurses are often the most effective and relevant communicators in the primary care team, and sometimes also the most effective diagnosticians (Iliffe 2000). That effectiveness is arguably a result of the fact that however overextended nursing theory may be, nursing knowledge and skills centre around an identifiable zone that is at the heart of the patient's own perceived experience and awareness. It is arguable also that the focus of nursing ethics and values connect well with the focus of nursing knowledge and skills. The professional commitment of nursing is to the health, care, well-being, autonomy and dignity of the individual patient, and the ethics and values of nursing focus precisely on that zone. In this respect we can see a profession that is consistent and coherent in its professional culture.

Deficits in the nursing repertoire

However, there are problems in this picture. I said earlier that nurses are the largest professional group in health care. They are also, from the patient's point of view, the key providers of care at the personal level, concerned with those aspects of the patient's life that the patient will see as central to their sense of self. They are therefore in a key position to shape the impact of health care. However, their individualistic focus also acts to disable them from fulfilling their potential as shapers of health care. The fact is that much of the work of developing health care does not take place at the patient's side, but in other places, and these places tend not to be those where the nurse is most comfortable. Health care is an activity undertaken in organisations of various sizes and constructions, and its operation is shaped by political agendas within those organisations and within the wider context of state, government and other stakeholders. Health care is increasingly seen as a response to social and economic issues, particularly to socio-economic inequality. It is increasingly involved in responding to the wider effects of social and cultural change as the bonds of social obligation and identity weaken. The health care system in the UK is a huge communal asset subject to intense competition in respect of its resources, and the professions involved all seek to exert influence over the use of that asset. The nursing profession is one of those involved, and whether nurses wish for this or not, they are engaged in the process of competition for influence.

It is in this situation where the present profile of the nursing profession in terms of its focus of values and knowledge-base becomes an issue. The wider social and economic concerns of health care planners require the application of perspectives that take account of collective as well as individual issues. Any organised group in this arena with a sense of its own interests and ideals needs to have a clear framework of political principles to enable it to convert these into realistic and acceptable goals. At present nursing lacks this. An interesting contrast can be made with the medical profession, which appears on the basis of its code of ethics to be every bit as individualistic as nurses in its moral orientation. However, doctors have developed other perspectives, which enable them to work with collective issues, while still apparently maintaining an individualistic stance. Other groups in health care are also equipped with their own principles that allow them to navigate through areas outside of direct patient care. The value-base of social work includes principles that are relevant to collective issues, primarily based on a political analysis of the distribution of power in society and a conception of social rights and equality. Again these allow social workers to engage confidently in debate with others in heath care on issues of policy and priorities beyond the requirements of specific patients.

By contrast, as Browne (2001) points out, nurses are characterised by their individualistic perspective. Interventions by nurses in policy debates in health care, while often well argued and forceful, tend to be undermined by the fact that they are not part of a deeper nursing perspective, and that it is therefore difficult to build up a consistent nursing case in relation to those issues, reflecting the values and aspirations of the profession. Clearly the development of such a case will not on its own render nurses more influential in the development of health care than they are at present. But coherence and consistency of ideas helps to focus the potential of nurses' central role in care, and of their numbers. As Kuhse (1997) suggests, nursing is a 'slumbering giant' in political terms, and needs to develop a shared political stance and strategy expressing the values of the profession.

Potential areas of influence

There are clearly identifiable areas where the potential exists for a major role for nursing, if the profession can develop a focused nursing perspective. One such area is the allocation of resources and the identification of priorities in health care. In 1948 and for decades afterward there was a general public assumption that the NHS was reactive to need and that the decision as to whose need justified the use of resources was a decision for doctors. The medical profession was trusted to deal with this on clinical criteria. Now there is wider awareness that resources fall short of need and that the question of who gets a particular treatment and who (individually or collectively) does not, is not one that can be resolved by doctors on clinical criteria alone. Although there is still a desire among the public for the decision to be taken by someone other than themselves, that is a symptom of confusion rather than consensus. Historically nurses have on the whole distanced themselves from the business of prioritising and rationing, and to a degree this is still the case. Degeling *et al.* (2000) have shown that British nurses remain uncomfortable with resource issues, and with the kind of rational decision-making that is necessary in this area. Interestingly they found Australian nurses to be more oriented toward these areas. An absolute commitment to the individual patient does not sit easily with any involvement in rationing and prioritising, as Nortvedt (2001) argues. It is therefore understandable that nurses have avoided this territory. However, I shall argue later in the book that such a stance is no longer viable, that involvement in rationing and prioritising is unavoidable for any group that wishes to influence health care.

There are other areas where the present state of affairs is uncertain, and where nursing may have an important role if it is able to develop an appropriate focus. An example of this is the evolution of organisations in health care, in the context of cultural and organisational change generally. Organisational change has been periodic in the NHS, but the frequency of major change has increased during its lifetime. Meanwhile in the outside world, our perception of organisations has evolved significantly in the past half-century. On the one hand, there is a greater awareness that organisations can be agents in their own right, and can exhibit behaviour that is more than the sum of the behaviour of the people working within them. On the other hand, there is a changing perception of the contingent nature of organisations, and a post-modern perspective that views organisations as social constructs, constantly changing and reconstituting.

These apparently contradictory perspectives on organisations operate to produce a situation where organisations are both important and highly problematic. The reality of most bureaucracy in modern societies is that organisations are constantly remaking themselves, or being remade, and are therefore in a permanent state of flux and uncertainty, which typically offers both threats and opportunities to those involved. Although most nurses work in organisations – often very large – there is an absence of an organisational perspective in nursing culture, ethics and theory. Many nurses become managers in such organisations, and unquestionably have built up a large body of experiential wisdom about organisational issues. But this does not seem to have produced a significant shift in the centre of gravity of nursing values, ethics or even politics toward an organisational focus. In particular there is very little systematic addressing of the issues that arise for a member of a code-regulated profession in taking a position of power in an organisation. This is a crucial experience in modern health care, and it is predominantly a nursing experience. Hewison (2001) has recently offered a relatively optimistic perspective on the potential of nurse managers to come into their own in this context, and to offer a creative melding of professional and organisation values. On the other hand, the persistent individualism of nursing thinking in the organisational context shows itself in Laurent's (2000) attempt to import an individualistic nursing model into the organisational context. The development of systems such as clinical governance which mix the legitimising features of professional and organisational structures ensure that this is an issue of pressing relevance.

Nurses are not unique in the above respects. Though many doctors have important organisational roles and considerable skills in this area, the organisational perspective has not found its way into the culture, ethics or even knowledge base of medicine. One sector of medicine, general practice, has relatively little organisational experience, and GPs as a group are probably less experienced in organisational issues than are nurses, given the structure of their work until recently. This will doubtless change as the new arrangements in primary care operate, and there is no obvious way that nursing culture and values will enable nurses to take a lead here. To do so would involve a considerable cultural change. But the situation is at present fluid, and open to being shaped by a group with a clear agenda.

Conclusion

Though nursing has some inherited disadvantages, both in terms of its external power-relations and in terms of its internal resources, it nonetheless has potential to play an increased role in the development of health care. Opportunities for change exist, but these belong to particular historical circumstances, which will not last for ever. So the opportunities may be lost. Two important areas discussed above where a nursing agenda needs to develop – organisational change and rationing – will each form the subject-matter of a subsequent chapter, and the possible shape of a new consensus will be further explored together with the potential role of nursing in the development of these.

3 Nursing and the state

Introduction

This chapter explores the relationship between nursing, state and government. The role of the state is briefly considered in the context of political theory, as is also the relationship between state and government. This is applied to the involvement of state and government in health care, and the principles that shape and justify this involvement. The discussion also outlines the political implications of a lack of consensus on fundamental moral principles, and the response to this problem offered by Rawls. Finally the mechanisms that link the state and government to the nursing profession are explored, together with the moral and political implication of this relationship for nursing.

Three relationships

In the United Kingdom three separate relationships connect the nursing profession and the state. In the first of these relationships the state acts as ultimate guarantor of the professional standards of nursing, through the legislation creating the UKCC and subsequently the Nursing and Midwifery Council. The old title 'state registered nurse' symbolised that relationship. The second relationship is that of employer and employee, and is based on the role of the state in the provision of health care. In the UK most health care is delivered through state-controlled organisations, and most nurses are employed by those organisations, so the state stands in the role of employer to most nurses.

These two relationships tell us something about the role of the state in health care. The first represents the regulatory role, involving the creation of a framework of rules and requirements that providers of health care must adhere to. This is a role taken by the state in all advanced societies. The second relationship involves the state acting directly in the provider role. This is a not a role that is taken by the state to the same degree or in the same way in all advanced societies. In the UK the state's role is particularly prominent, and therefore has a more direct impact on the work of nurses than would be the case in the United States. The dual relationship that exists in the UK means that the nursing profession must relate to the state, both as professionals, with regard to the maintenance of standards, and as employees, with regard to pay and working conditions.

I mentioned three relationships, but have only discussed two so far. In the third relationship nurses relate to the state – or more properly to the government – as an interest group seeking to influence health policy. This constitutes a rather different kind of relationship from the first two in that nursing, as one of the stakeholders of the health care system, must actively seek to maintain some influence over the running of that system. A good deal more will be said about this relationship in Chapter 8, but for the moment we must consider the nature of the other partners in these relationships, the state and the government.

State and government

State and government are often merged into one entity in health-related discussions, but this conceals important distinctions. In modern political systems the term 'state' is generally applied to the collection of institutions that focuses legitimate political authority within a set of internationally recognised national frontiers. Usually this will include legislature, executive and judiciary, together with civil service, police and military, and the machinery for a range of state provisions. There are several models of the state, but we only need be concerned with two of these. One of the dominant models in terms of contemporary political culture in the western world is the liberal state. In most versions of this model the state is a somewhat passive institutional framework that does not seek to pursue a particular set of goals or values, and has no agenda other than to maintain itself and perform its functions. However, that is not to say that the thinking behind the liberal state is neutral and value-free. On the contrary, according to Gray (1995) traditional liberal political theory places special value on liberty, and as Schwartzmantel (1994) points out in his discussion of the liberal state, liberalism at its most uncompromising views the state as a necessary evil, on the basis that states have an innate tendency to interfere with individual liberty if permitted. The state should not only be neutral and passive but also minimal in its activities, confining itself to maintaining law, order and defence from outside aggression. For other provisions, including education and health care, the traditional liberal would doubt the suitability of the state as a provider.

The liberal model of the state makes a clear distinction between state and government, in that whereas the state as a whole is neutral and passive, government is an active element within the state apparatus, usually seen as centring on the executive and legislature. Government can legitimately represent a particular set of political principles, and have an active agenda. In the liberal model, action by the state is in many cases really action by the government. It is important to bear in mind that liberal states do not have to be democratic. The model does not dictate the exact way governments shall be selected, though it requires that they be selected in a way that is consistent and constitutional. However, when the contemporary liberal state is discussed, the assumption is usually made that it is a liberal *democratic* state, where governments are selected in accordance with the will of the people, and the constitution of the state expresses the principle of popular sovereignty.

The other model of the state relevant to our concerns is the statist model. This model developed out of the liberal democratic dilemma identified by Schwartzmantel and is a response to the problem of the popular will in liberal democracies requiring the state to take a more active role in the lives of citizens than the liberal state would permit. Statists argue that this active role is legitimate, that the will of the people ought to be expressed through state institutions and that governments have a legitimate role in creating and using state institutions for this purpose. The statist model developed momentum through much of the twentieth century, as the state itself expanded its role in response to war, economic problems and social pressures (Cronin 1991).

The principle of state involvement was developed, particularly by social democrats, during the early twentieth century, and was expressed in the UK in the creation of the welfare state in the 1940s. The way this was done helps to highlight the distinction between state and government. The welfare state, a complex of state institutions providing health care, social care, education and income maintenance, was the creation of specific governments, but a significant part of the machinery of that welfare state was run by organisations which government could not normally control on a day-to-day basis. These were far from being simply extensions of the bureaucracy of government, and in many cases had a clear corporate identity, in law or in fact. The distinction between state and government helps to make sense of this situation. The welfare state became in a real sense part of the machinery of the state, but is not in the same sense part of the machinery of government.

The other way in which the statist model differs from the liberal model of the state is that the statist accepts the use of the state by government and people to promote political and moral principles other than liberty. The social democratic governments of Europe in the twentieth century have sought to remould state institutions to express the values of equality and social solidarity, attaching a social democratic programme to the liberal state and creating what Cronin terms the 'liberal socialist state'. The British National Health Service is a particularly interesting example of this process, as according to Johnson and Cullen (2000) its creation expressed precisely those two values I have mentioned, equality and social solidarity. However, its operation has tended to express rather different values. I discuss this further later in the chapter.

The state and health care

The salient fact in the politics of health care in the UK since 1979 has been the tension between the statist principles of the welfare state, and the renewed interest in the liberal model of the state within the conservative party which came into office in that year under Margaret Thatcher's leadership. The Thatcher government sought to reduce the role of the state throughout British society, and to achieve a significant shift back toward the original model of the liberal state. In other areas – particularly in the nationalised industries – this was achieved by a return to private ownership, removing the state from direct involvement. However, in health care the conservative reforms did not focus on privatisation but rather on decentralisation from large bodies at regional and district level, to smaller bodies, in particular to NHS trusts. Bartlett and LeGrand (1994: p. 55) call these 'independent non-governmental organisations', but they remain part of the state system, not least because they are directly accountable to the secretary of state. However, they are smaller in scale, more local, more autonomous, and less state-like in the traditional sense than the old NHS. A similar process happened in education, where schools were enabled to opt out of local authority control. The government's expectation was that bodies such as NHS trusts and opted-out schools would, because of their scale and their relationship to other bodies, behave less like state bodies and more like private bodies, with a flexible market-oriented approach. In a sense the conceptual boundary between state and private activity was blurred. Even though these bodies are still part of the state system, the hope of their creators was that their culture and behaviour would be less state-like. What is clear is that the autonomy of these decentralised bodies allowed the government to divest itself of some accountability for their operation while, as Light (2001) points out, gaining a good deal in terms of real control. So what has happened is not that the role of the state has been reduced, but that the relationship between state and government has shifted, with central government differently involved in the running of the welfare state.

Since the return of the labour party to government in 1997 there has been only a modest return to statist principles. Part of the conceptual shift toward the liberal model of the state has become established across much of the political spectrum, and there is greater scepticism about ability of government and state to achieve major social outcomes among all major political parties than there was thirty years ago. However, health care remains largely a state provision, and we need to consider what principles underpin and justify the involvement of the state in the provision of that particular good.

In Chapter 1, I considered the moral significance of health and the moral justifications for providing health care. I also considered briefly the justifications for government involvement in health care provision. We now need to consider this further, and I start by considering equality of access to health care as one of the justifications of state involvement. The concept of equality draws from the idea of equality of intrinsic worth between individuals, an idea deeply rooted in Kantian ethics, wherein equality is based on shared personhood; and also from utilitarianism where the formula 'each counts for one and none for more than one' is a fundamental principle in establishing the benefits, and therefore the morality, of an action. That equality of worth does not manifest in ordinary daily living, where disparities of luck and talent lead to very unequal outcomes both in terms of economic success and of health. Economic inequalities may be acceptable as a by-product of freedom, but as the Commission on Social Justice (1994) argued, where these inequalities involve an inability of some people to meet basic needs this may be seen as a more fundamental threat to that intrinsic equality of worth and to carry no counterbalancing justifications in relation to individual freedom. We might extend the idea of basic needs to such areas as a reasonable life-expectancy and the ability to protect oneself from disease. Only the state can ensure that every citizen has equal access to a particular good. (Incidentally that does not mean that the state has to provide it directly, only that it has to have ultimate control of that provision.) So this is a legitimate arena for state involvement. Taking the Kantian justification a little further, it is clear that the equality of worth based on shared personhood links closely to the requirement of autonomy as something equally required by all persons. Social inequality is justified largely because it is the product of individual freedom, and this justification can only make sense in terms of distributive justice if that freedom is itself equally distributed, so that we start on a level playing field. Freedom is about the ability to take opportunities, and justice requires that freedom be equally distributed. So, Daniels (1985) argues from the principle of 'fair equality of opportunity' that health care ought to be equally available in order that, in a competitive society, everyone is playing on that same level playing field.

However, there are also other principles expressed by state involvement in health care. Prominent among these is solidarity, the principle that the community ought to provide support to its members even when that support cannot be reciprocated. This can be argued from the same bases as the principle of equal access, that is the equality of worth of each member of the community.

Such equality justifies mutual aid because it implies recognition of the intrinsic worth of each community member. But it also draws from a different, collectivist tradition of thinking which views the self-sufficient individual is an illusion and argues that everyone is dependent on the community for their identity and their survival. Mutual aid is a legitimate and deeply rooted part of community life, but in modern societies, runs the argument, neither the individual nor the community have the resources to mobilise the goods necessary for survival. Only the state is in a position to do this. This again is not necessarily an argument for state provision, but could justify state initiative and direction, and many have argued that it is a better expression of social solidarity if the state facilitates and promotes health care provision within the community, rather than acting as the direct provider. By doing this, commentators such as Green (1999) argue, the state avoids the situation where community solidarity is sapped by dependence on state provision.

Another justification for state involvement in health care is based on the utilitarian principle of maximising well-being. The outline of this philosophy was set out in Chapter 2, but its relevance here is clear. The legitimacy of liberal and statist states rests on the ability to justify their existence rationally, and the strongest rational justification is that such states benefit their citizens. A state does not have much point if it does no good. Ryan (1991: p. 94) expresses the utilitarian view of the state as follows: 'the state exists to do whatever good it can, so all states are welfare states'. So we can argue that it is legitimate to apply the utilitarian test to the activity of the state as to the actions of an individual. It is important to note here that the utilitarian does not assume that the principles of solidarity and equality necessarily serve to maximise well-being. Even if an egalitarian and solidaristic national health service produces a preponderance of well-being over ill-being, that is not enough for the utilitarian. The utilitarian requires that the state's provision of health care achieves the best out of all the available options in terms of maximising well-being. For a particular state health care system to be justified on utilitarian grounds, it must offer the most productive use of those particular resources. And that may conflict with solidarity and equality.

In different ways the traditional biomedical areas of health care and the more recent developments of health promotion both

present difficulties for the utilitarian in evaluating the contribution of health care to the health of the population served. It is
by no means obvious in either case that health care in the form
offered, or indeed health care at all, is the best way to maximise
health. The health benefits of good housing and good education
are strongly suggested by the available evidence on health inequalities, where the lack of these items is associated with poor health.
Should we not consider the relative benefits of spending our money
on those benefits, rather than on health care? If we are concerned
primarily with well-being we might discover, as Oliver (2001)
points out, that increasing expenditure on health care is not the
most effective way of maximising well-being. The utilitarian justification, if applied rigorously, may not lead us to support the
existing state provision of health care.

Principles of the NHS in 1948

We have, then, a set of principles that provide a base for state and
government involvement in health care. We need to consider now
the principles that can be identified in the structure and functioning of the National Health Service as it has developed over half a
century. A number of conscious choices were made in the 1940s,
which determined the shape of the NHS, and these all provide
useful indications as to the values underlying its creation. It is clear
from the way the system was set up that it was intented to achieve
equal access to health care. In practice this was not achieved because of pre-existing regional and district inequalities in the hospital system, but the provision of health care free at the point of
use sought to ensure that inequalities of income had no impact at
any stage on access to care. However, the British system was and
remains a 'gatekeeper' system, wherein access to services is exten-
sively controlled by one gatekeeper, the general practitioner. The
GP decides what treatment or care the patient should have, and
patients cannot in practice easily 'shop around' among GPs. So,
the patient's scope for autonomous choice is very limited indeed.
It is clear from this that whereas the principle of equality was
strongly enshrined in the structure of the NHS, the principle of
patient autonomy was given little weight. We might say that the
equality embodied in the system was an expression of the equality

of collective solidarity, rather than of the equality of autonomous personhood. This accords with Klein's (1995) comment that the view of health as a social good tended to be stronger in the planning process than the view of health as an individual right.

The structure of the NHS as set up in 1948 also expressed an interestingly ambiguous position on the value of democracy. Community health care was placed in the remit of the local authorities, democratically elected bodies accountable to their local electorates. Hospital services were put under the control of local and regional boards appointed rather than elected and dominated by hospital-based consultants. This may look at first sight like a system balanced between democracy and paternalism. However, in 1948 and for decades afterwards health care in the UK was dominated by hospital medicine, in terms of resources, power and prestige. In 1948 community health care was undoubtedly in second place in all these respects. So paternalism triumphed, because it determined the fate of the most important areas of health care as they were perceived at the time. This balance of power arose partly out of the process of negotiation. The medical profession was strongly opposed to local authority control of hospitals. But Klein (1995) suggests that Bevan was himself motivated by the values of paternalistic rationalism, propelling him toward equality, efficiency and uniformity and away from the local democracy and flexibility of a local authority-based system. By the 1970s the balance of importance between hospital and community care was beginning to change, and recognition of the significance of primary care and community health care was gaining ground. So it is interesting that in 1974 local authorities lost most of their community health functions to unelected health authorities, which were the direct descendants of the 1948 hospital authorities. Overall we can say that from 1948 to the present, central government and its advisors have consistently chosen not to entrust the key parts of the health care system to democratically elected bodies other than central government itself. In that respect Bevan set a pattern that has been consistently maintained.

It can be argued that the NHS as constructed in 1948 did in fact fit well with the society that it served. Despite the upsurge of democratic and egalitarian principles expressed in the Labour victory of 1945, British society and culture were nonetheless, as Jones (1997) points out, still profoundly unequal. So it need not be surprising that paternalism tempered equality in the creation of the NHS. The dominance of a high status group like the medical profession makes sense in that context. The pursuit of efficiency and uniformity can also be understood historically. British society in 1948 was perceived by most of its members as being homogenous, with a strong base of shared beliefs and values, and common goals and aspirations. This view had a significant impact on perceptions as to what a national health service should provide, as health care needs were seen as consistent across the population, and best met by a service that was geared to homogenous, efficient mass-provision.

Principles of the NHS since 1948

In many respects the NHS in 1948 could be seen as an example of a 'fordist' institution. This term denotes the institutions and processes that emerged in the early part of the century to serve a mass-market, the paradigm case of which is the motor industry and the Model T Ford. The application of the concept to health care is developed by writers such as Walby and Greenwell (1994) in the UK context and by Navarro (1994) in the US context. The fordist organisation works on the assumption that its mission is to supply a homogenous market, serving as many people as possible as efficiently as possible by offering a standardised product. Whilst fordism is egalitarian it is also paternalistic and conformist. The fordist mode of production and consumption has been argued to be the distinguishing characteristic of the early-to-mid-twentieth century economy and society. Serious cracks in fordist conformity appeared in the cultural upheavals in the western world in the 1960s. While deeper social change eroded the general faith in a consensus-based society that had obtained in the 1940s and the '50s, later economic problems eroded the political consensus between the major parties that had existed from the early 1950s, a consensus that involved the centre-left and centre-right both accepting the need for a welfare state. After the economic crises of the 1960s governments sought means of managing the health service in a more proactive way, to control costs and achieve rational planning. However, deteriorating economic circumstances in the 1970s increased pressure considerably, and in 1979 a conservative government, determined to reduce public spending, put an end to political consensus. A renewed attempt to increase efficiency by the introduction of general managers in the 1980s was followed by a corporate decentralisation in 1990, which constituted the most significant change since 1948.

The problems of the Thatcher government in reforming the NHS are highly instructive in considering the difficulties of running a system built upon consensus when that consensus has broken down. Despite that government's privatising agenda in other sectors, it felt unable to privatise health care, not least because the electorate were deeply attached to the NHS. And although the government was keen to enhance the individual citizen's economic role as a consumer, it had no particular desire to empower the citizen in other ways, certainly not in any way that smacked of collectivism. Local democracy was not on the whole well-regarded in the Thatcher government, so there was no attempt to democratise the NHS by linking it to elected bodies. It is clear that the government wanted to enhance patient autonomy by emphasising individual responsibility for health. This was done through health promotion policies, particularly those promulgated in *The Health of the Nation* (Department of Health 1992a); and also through the introduction of the consumer role into health care, embodied in *The Patient's Charter* (Department of Health 1992b). However, this was only achieved in a very limited way, because the government was also committed to controlling costs. The gatekeeper role of the GP was not only retained, but also enhanced, with the result that the patient gained little in terms of initiative and autonomy. The GP remained in control of the patient's access to the service.

It is clear, then that these apparently extensive changes did not achieve a real change in the underlying priorities of the NHS. Despite its anti-egalitarian stance in general, the conservative government did not in a fundamental way attack the egalitarian intention of the NHS. Inequalities were exacerbated, but this was largely accidental, resulting from the patchy introduction of reforms such as GP fundholding, which created inequalities in terms of practice and locality (Bain 1994). Despite the government's commitment to individual autonomy in general, patient autonomy was not greatly enhanced. And despite its generally radical agenda the government felt unable to privatise health care. They judged, no doubt accurately, that they had no mandate to do this and, that there was no immediate prospect of a new consensus developing that would accommodate private health care on a mass scale. There is no question that there was a cultural change in the direction of greater individualism in British and other western societies, and that the Thatcher government both benefited from it and promoted it. This individualism has shown itself in a range of social changes concerning work, family and community life. But in the late 1980s it was not comprehensive or deep enough to effect the attitudinal change necessary to support privatisation of the health service. Nor, probably, has it become so in the early 2000s. So what the reforms of 1990 produced was a different way of structuring state health care to make it more cost-effective.

The 1997 labour government has re-reformed this system, but has not departed greatly from the underlying structural principles. Primary care has been reorganised to be more similar to the rest of the system, and its relative importance has been enhanced. Arguably this increases further the power of GPs, and again challenges the power of hospital consultants. But patient autonomy is not further enhanced, and the inequality of power between patient and doctor remains. Despite a commitment to the idea of civil society, and a flirtation with communitarianism, the 1997 labour government has retained the principle that all NHS bodies are state bodies, ultimately accountable to the government.

It remains to be seen whether the changes of the late 1990s will succeed in adapting the priorities of health care to contemporary society, and effectively move away from the fordist principles of 1948. The last two governments have both created an expectation that they would remodel the health care system in accordance with their ideology, but it is not clear that they have in fact done so. In each case they have left much of their predecessor's work intact. As Powell (2000) points out, claims to have created a new NHS seem exaggerated in both cases. Neither government has noticeably succeeded in using the NHS as an instrument for achieving significant change in the wider society. In that respect, Bevan retains the prize.

Government values and health

What should be the proper relationship between the government and the NHS? What values and principles should guide governments in their running of the NHS? During the twentieth century governments of the right and left have often claimed a clear ideological and moral agenda, purporting to provide an equally clear choice for the electorate. However, there is a shift in recent decades toward an acknowledgement that the power of democratic governments to remould society in accordance with their ideology is very limited. In the view of commentators such as Held (1995) the increasingly complex and global nature of key institutions makes the power of individual governments more limited as time passes. Much of the time governments react to events and struggle to make small incremental steps to larger goals. The retreat of tribal party loyalty and a tendency toward more calculated decisions by the electorate identified by Giddens (1998) encourages governments to follow, rather than lead public opinion. This could be seen as indicative of a deterioration in the political culture, but it can equally be seen as a rational response to a changing situation. In the case of the NHS, the values of democracy are surely served if the government seeks to reflect public concerns and priorities in its running of health care.

The problem with following rather than leading public opinion is that public concerns and priorities are neither consistent nor universal. In a diverse multicultural society there is often no consensus on major issues. So government cannot depend on public opinion to provide guidance that is consistent and considered. So what are governments to do, if party loyalties and ideologies are not robust enough to give guidance? One liberal view of contemporary western society, expressed in particular by Rawls (1993), suggests that there is no sustainable common view of the good life, and that no such view ought to be reflected by the state, which ought to be neutral on fundamental moral issues. However, this view has been contested by a number of writers, including Kymlicka (2000), who argues that it is impossible for liberal states to be neutral in terms of values or culture. Clearly it makes little sense to say that particular governments can have no moral stance whatsoever, but the real issue is how far government should seek to embody its stance in the apparatus of the state. This issue presents real problems for contemporary British government in relation to the NHS. As I have already suggested, the NHS is far from neutral in terms of the values it embodies, and it has proved difficult for governments – even those with strong ideological agendas – to significantly change its direction. And yet it is impossible for government actions with regard to the NHS to be in any real sense neutral. What should a government do?

I suggested in Chapter 1 that health is a value, similar in some ways to other values such as wisdom, beauty and happiness and that it has a real degree of universality. However, descriptive definitions of health vary between cultures, and also vary a good deal within a diverse society like that of Britain. It is inevitable that government will be involved in the promotion of health, and we can see dangers in a government imposing a particular, perhaps partial version of health on society. Commentators on Health Promotion such as O'Brien (1995) have identified this danger in recent years. On the other hand, it is difficult for anyone to seek or promote health if they hold no beliefs of their own about what constitutes health. Rawls (1993) encounters the same issue with the concept of justice, a moral principle derivable from fundamental definitions of the good. Rawls sees justice as a necessary component of a workable political system. He avoids the problem of the state imposing a partial notion of justice on citizens who operate from a different morality, by introducing the concept of overlapping consensus. He argues that it is possible to support a common definition of justice from several quite different moralities. Though the 'territory' covered by different moralities may in large part be very different, there can be some overlap also, and overlap in crucial areas can provide the basis for a stable political order in otherwise very diverse societies. Can something similar be achieved with health? In Chapter 1, I suggested that there is some overlap between different definitions of health, though it is not clear whether such overlap is deep or wide enough to provide legitimacy or stability for particular models of health care.

Nurses and the state

The applicability and viability of the idea of overlapping consensus to health care is explored further in Chapter 7. At this point I shall confine myself to considering some preliminary issues concerning the role of nurses in this situation. To do this I shall step back a little and revisit the different relationships between nurses, government and the state, which I touched on early in this chapter. I identified a regulatory role for the state in setting up and sustaining the UKCC, and subsequently the NMC, as part of the apparatus of professional regulation. There are two models for this role. One is for the state to perform a minimal, neutral role, keeping the wheels of the system turning and providing for basic safely and security. The other is for the state to support a particular set of values through its support of the profession. We can see the work of bodies such as the NMC as explicitly value-laden, in terms of the requirements they lay upon nurses. Neither their codes of conduct nor their procedures are neutral in value terms. But we might ask how far these values carry the imprimatur of the state, and how far this is simply a matter of a profession regulating itself, making use of essentially neutral state apparatus. The answer to this might vary depending on our model of the state. If we incline to the liberal model, we will expect, or desire, a neutral state holding the ring for the nursing profession to operate effectively. If we incline toward the statist model we would expect, or desire, a state which is more actively engaged in supporting the values of nursing and seeking to ensure that its values are represented within nursing.

There is another framework of analysis that we can bring in to illuminate further the state-nursing relationship. That is the idea of the contract. May (1975) argued that regulatory bodies (he was concerned with medicine) represent a contractual relationship between state, patient and professional, and Chadwick and Tadd (1992) consider the same model in relation to the UKCC. The legislation setting up the UKCC and the NMC can be seen as statements of commitment on the part of the state to a particular role for the nursing profession. The code of professional conduct can be seen as a statement of commitment by the nursing profession to practice in certain ways. They are in a real sense two sides of a moral contract between profession and state. On registration every nurse 'signs up' to the nursing side of the contract. Every government is committed to its side of the contract, until it chooses to change the legislation and therefore change the contract. Governments are acting, in part, on behalf of the population, in entering into that contract. So in another sense the contract is also between the individual nurse and the individual patient, with NMC and government acting as agents of the two parties. Whether we are liberal or statist in our view of the state, the idea of the contract gives a firmer moral base to this relationship between the state and the nursing profession, and a model also of the nurse-patient relationship.

However, the NMC also represents part of the labour government's agenda of modernising professional regulation (Department of Health 2000) and its operation may bring about a shift in relationships. In particular, it has more patient and stakeholder representation than did the UKCC, and ostensibly a more accountable relationship with the public (Department of Health 2001). In these respects the government is seeking to embody its values into the operation of this body, in a way that was much less apparent in the case of the UKCC. These values include equality, openness and inclusion. This approach certainly accords with a statist view of the relationship discussed above. It may be that the change of representation will also change the contractual relationship somewhat, in that the public, instead of relying on government to represent them through its oversight of the UKCC, will be more directly represented on the NMC, alongside other bodies. The long-term effects of this are hard to predict, but it may mean that the new body will not so easily be able to represent nursing to other bodies, but will instead to some degree constitute a forum in which nursing's relationships with the public, the NHS and other stakeholders, are negotiated.

I also identified a relationship between the state and nurses as employees. In that role nurses have experienced little of the neutral state in recent years. Just as there was nothing neutral about the setting up of the NHS – with all the implications for nurses' conditions of employment that followed from this – so there was nothing neutral about the changes brought into the system in the 1980s and the 1990s, in their impact on nurses' working lives. Here we see the state, not as a neutral structure, but as an instrument of government ideology. In particular, the conservative government's priority of economy and efficiency in the 1980s and the early '90s expressed wider values about the state and economy, and, as Wells (1999) points out, impacted considerably on the way nurses worked. This created pressures that called into question the balance between professional and the employee roles, and the appropriate priority of loyalties. So the nurse-state relationship in this context was one in which government values were imposed on the state system and on nurses within it. For these reasons the nurse's recent experience of the state as employer involves a rather more disempowering relationship than the experience of professional regulation through state institutions.

The third relationship which I identified at the beginning of the chapter, that of stakeholder in the health care system, is not really with the state at all, but with government. This involves the nursing profession engaging with the government and other bodies in negotiating the shape of health care. In order to fulfil this role, nursing needs to retain a degree of separateness from government, and also from the state, so that a distinctive nursing agenda can be developed and included in debate. I think it follows from my argument so far that government cannot be passive in developing an appropriate health care system, and that the process of developing and negotiating a consensus on health and health care requires government involvement. However, it cannot depend on government to bear fruit. Other institutions need to be involved also, and those with the most inclusive and flexible view of health and health care have most to offer in this. This makes nursing a particularly important participant in this process. The process of consensus-building must be characterised by relationships of equality, and those with the greatest ability to accommodate a range of views at a level of equality are likely to be most effective in this process. The nursing approach to health and health care is more inclusive, more flexible and less hierarchical than the approach of the other main likely participants – particularly the government, civil service and medical profession. At the same time nursing ethics retains a traditional focus on the concept of duty, which anchors it to a secure value base. In all these respects nursing has major advantages in contributing to consensus-building, through their ability to communicate on common ground with the widest range of perspectives.

Conclusion

The history of the relationships between nursing and the state has been shaped by the evolution of nursing and likewise the evolution of the state's role in health care. Although not static, these relationships have provided a stable point of reference for the nursing profession. However, recent and ongoing changes in government policy are changing the parameters of those relationships in a way that offers major opportunities for nursing.

4 Nursing and the citizen

Introduction

This chapter explores the relationship between the nurse and the patient in terms of its moral and political significance. In order to develop this theme, the idea of citizenship and the implications of this for the individual citizen are discussed in relation to the state and to other citizens. Some of the links that connect the citizen to the nurse are considered, together with the significance of those connections.

Citizenship

Universal citizenship is essentially a modern concept that evolved with the development of democratic ideas in the eighteenth century. As Delanty (2000) makes clear, the ancient idea of citizenship was anything but universal, and applied only to the free and enfranchised members of small communities. Citizens in that context were generally a minority, and operated as a ruling class, dominating a subject population of free foreigners, women and slaves. Citizenship as a universal status was established in practice first in the late eighteenth century, in the series of constitutions drawn up by the legislatures of the United States and France in the years after their respective revolutions. This version of citizenship was closely dependent on the development of ideas of political democracy and popular sovereignty in those societies. The concept was widely adopted in Europe and Latin America as those continents went through revolutionary upheavals inspired by the American and French examples. Since then the concept of citizenship has been associated with democratic constitutional government throughout the world.

The modern idea of citizenship is rooted in a concept of human worth and human equality that developed particularly in the philosophy of Immanuel Kant and the political theory of John Locke. The concept is paradoxical in that it is universal, as an expression of the equal worth of all human beings, but at the same time it is the particular expression of that universal idea. Citizenship is associated with the state, and legally to be a citizen one must be a citizen of a specific state. Usually (although not always) citizenship of one state precludes citizenship of others. So the role of citizen has a duality arising from this situation. Citizenship on one level denotes liberty and empowerment; but it also implied a degree of dependence, in that the status can only be assumed in the context of a particular state. Citizenship is in a sense a resource, which can be used as leverage by the individual against the state but also by the state against the individual. The other point to note is that citizenship is a concept which only the liberal and statist models of the state can truly accommodate. Citizenship developed alongside, as an inextricable part of, the liberal state, and a large part of the liberal state's function is to ensure that its activities do not limit the liberty of the citizen.

The early-to-mid twentieth century saw a major critique and revision of the liberal model of citizenship. One of its best-known critics, T. H. Marshall (1950) argued that citizenship has evolved beyond the liberal principle of non-interference in the citizen's liberty, and that citizen's rights characteristic of the liberal state, which he termed civil rights, were only part of what was required in the modern state. To these he added political rights (the right to vote etc.), which I have identified with the liberal *democratic* state. He also added social rights (to health and social care) to the list. These last, in particular, helped to provide the basis for the social democratic model of citizenship, and of the state, in which the state actively seeks to promote the welfare of the citizen. More recently as O'Brien and Penna (1998) argue, citizenship has come to be seen on the political left as extending beyond social rights, to a point where it also requires social and cultural inclusion, and equality of esteem between different lifestyles and identities. However, the liberal view of citizenship, confined to the enjoyment of civil and political rights, remains strong on the political right wing, and was very much part of the Thatcherite vision.

In the United Kingdom the status of citizen is somewhat problematic even in civil and political terms. Faulks (1998) suggests that traditional constitutional usage has reflected the monarchical roots of the state, and the 'citizens' of the UK are, strictly speaking, subjects rather than citizens, leading to arguments that this has had the effect of perpetuating a deferential political culture and an excessively powerful executive. Despite the ambiguity of constitutional theory, the reality of citizenship is taken for granted by most inhabitants of the UK. However, constitutional guarantees of the rights of the citizen are taken in most such societies as a necessary underpinning of the citizen's status, and the absence of such guarantees in the UK can be seen as a problem.

Our particular concern in this chapter is to consider the moral and political basis of the relationship between the nurse and the patient. I shall work on the assumption that, whatever else they may be, all patients are citizens, and that they have that in common with all nurses. This does not mean that all patients, or all nurses, are British citizens, which is clearly not the case. It is rather to acknowledge that citizenship is the political and constitutional expression of the universal status, referred to often as personhood, which in Kantian ethics provides the basis for moral relations between human beings. I shall consider the relative significance of citizenship as against personhood as such. However, first we need to consider the relationship of citizens one to another, as nurses are fellow citizens with their patients, and this must form part of the bedrock of their relationship.

The moral basis of citizenship

In the liberal political tradition the basis of citizenship, as of personhood, is autonomy and rationality. Citizenship is predicated on the ability of the citizen to make rational choices in their actions and to take responsibility for their actions, a relationship which, according to Seligman (1993), owes a good deal to Kant. Kant's categorical imperative enjoined all rational persons to treat each other as members of a 'kingdom of ends' (Paton 1978); in other words, as part of a political community of rational beings who therefore have the ability to act rationally and are in that sense moral beings on an equal footing with one another. Kant's famous injunction not to treat purely as a means those who are ends sums up the moral heart of liberal thought. Exploitation of others, so they are used purely as a means to achieve our own ends, denies the personhood of those people and is also a denial of citizenship and a threat to a liberal polity. This does not rule out all actions involving the 'using' of another person, because any action involving another person through which we benefit ourselves in a sense involves such 'using'. We are all using one another all the time. The problem arises when the transaction is exclusively geared to the using of the other person, and their own autonomous interests are not regarded at all. Situations involving duress, deception and exploitation all deny the fact that the other person is also an 'end' because they prevent them from acting with full autonomy or with regard to their own interests.

It should be noted that these principles operate on the assumption of a balance between self-interest and duty. One assumption behind Kant's categorical imperative is that persons will seek their self-interest, rationally understood, and that morality is concerned with ensuring that opportunities to pursue our self-interest are properly distributed. The other influential ethical perspective, utilitarianism, is also based on the proposition that humans will seek their self-interest, (more specifically that they will seek pleasure, happiness or well-being, depending on which formulation we are using) and that morality must involve ensuring that as many people as possible are maximally enabled to pursue their self-interest and maximise their pleasure/happiness/well-being. Utilitarian and Kantian ethics, which are in many respects the most influential underpinnings to modern ethical theory in health care, carry an expectation that the pursuit of self-interest, undertaken rationally, is the most secure and sustainable basis for relationships between citizens. Selflessness and self-sacrifice are not part of the liberal moral framework for the citizen.

Citizen rights and duties

In considering the nurse-citizen interaction, we need to take account of the rights and duties of the citizen, as part of the moral landscape which the citizen inhabits. The citizen's rights arise from the moral status of the citizen, some of which depend in part on the moral status of the person. Miller (1976) divides rights generally into two kinds – those that we see as belonging intrinsically to human beings in general, irrespective of the political arrangements that surround them; and those that depend for their existence on the legal and political framework in force in that situation. The former are often termed human rights, or moral rights; the latter, positive rights. The recognition of human rights within a particular society can be translated into the establishing of positive rights into that legal system, which will in turn protect the citizen's human rights. As an example, the moral responsibility and autonomy of the citizen in Kantian ethics justifies recognition of a human right of the individual to determine her/his affairs. In both the liberal and the social democratic state this can in turn translate into positive rights, in this case legal and constitutional rights to freedom of movement, speech and association.

However, in other areas the liberal and social democratic views differ. I have outlined Marshall's framework of citizen's rights above, and it is clear that his concept of social rights, characteristic of a social democratic view of citizenship, are of a rather different kind from civil and (to a lesser degree) political rights. The existence of a right implies the existence of a duty on the part of another, in this case the state. Rights such as freedom of speech, movement and so on, require only that the state restrains itself from interference in the citizen's liberty. Political rights such as the right to vote involve some state bodies submitting themselves to the collective power of citizens, through elections. But social rights, such as rights to health and social care, involve a far more active role by the state, in mobilising and distributing material resources of various kinds for citizens. So, although these rights seemed to Marshall to form a logical continuity, they involve fundamentally different duties for the state.

The citizen's duties are generally less well defined than their rights. In the liberal model of the state the citizen's main duty is to respect the liberty of other citizens. This is normally achieved through the observance of the laws framed with this purpose in view, and also through the citizen's personal conduct toward fellow citizens. The citizen also has a duty to pay taxes, insofar as these are spent on safeguarding the citizen's liberty through law, order and national security. The liberal state's demands on the citizen are limited, and for many liberals the above is the complete list. For a social democrat, the state/citizen relationship is more complex, and might involve a number of actions that are geared not just to the liberty of fellow citizens but to their positive welfare. So, the payment of taxes will include an element for welfare provision as well as for the safeguarding of liberty. In reality however the social democrat view of the citizen's duty seems in many ways as anaemic and apologetic as that of the liberal. Plant (1992), arguing from a social democratic perspective, confines his list to the payment of taxes.

It is worth mentioning at this point that a third view exists which has been identified by several commentators (e.g. Mouffe 1993) as providing an alternative to the liberal and social democratic views of citizen duty. This perspective is known as civic republicanism, a political theory based on ancient city-state and renaissance models and eighteenth-century writers such as Rousseau, which accepts a limited, democratic state, but which identifies a number of specific duties on the part of the citizen, including one of political participation. The civic republican model of citizenship is accordingly a good deal more active than the liberal or social democratic models, and works on a much more positive and involved relationship between citizen and state. It also works on the assumption that active involvement in politics and in the life of the community and the republic generally will be in the citizen's interests, so the citizen's duty of participation does not require altruism or moral excellence, but the same kind of rational appreciation of self-interest that is required by liberalism.

Nurse, patient and citizen

In considering the nurse's role in relation to the patient, we need to take account of the same three levels that applied in relation to the nurse's relationship to the state. Nurses are professionals and the nursing profession is a significant social institution in most western societies. At the same time the nursing profession is a stakeholder in the health care system and a protagonist in the politics of health. Finally, nurses are employees, and have a relationship to their employers, which are mainly state and public bodies. Just as I suggested that the relationship between the nursing profession and the state has a contractual element to it, so, I would suggest, does the nurse-patient and nurse-citizen relationship. The nursing profession has a set of principles and values which, without being entirely consistent or unambiguous, are nonetheless relatively clear and clearly expressed at different levels of complexity. I have suggested that these can be taken as constituting an undertaking to behave in certain ways, in accordance with certain principles. This undertaking communicates itself to the state, or rather to the state's active agents, including the government. It also communicates itself to the citizen, and that includes the citizen in her or his more dependent role as patient. Clearly most citizens will not be familiar with the terms of nursing's code of profession conduct, although it is a public document and available for anyone to study. But the general ethos of nursing is communicated in a range of ways. Nurses as a profession have committed themselves to working to specific principles, and that commitment has major implications for their relationship with the patient/citizen.

The nurse and the rights of the citizen

The professional commitment of the nurse needs to relate to the rights and duties of the patient and others, in their role as citizen, and in their other roles. This leads immediately to a number of problems. First, the assumption of rationality, upon which the citizen role is based, clearly cannot be taken as applying to the behaviour of patients or their relatives, who in the stress of illness may behave irrationally. So the first dilemma for the nurse is to find a way between those two facts in her interaction with the patient. Clearly much in nursing practice and nursing ethics is geared to finding the right balance between responding to the rational autonomous citizen and responding to the dependent and often irrational patient. The emphasis in ethics literature written by nurses on informed consent and patient autonomy (e.g. White 1994) can be seen as an expression of commitment to sustain the citizen in the patient, because it is citizenship that provides the moral basis for informed consent. There is evidence that nurses in practice place a high priority on liberty, expressed as patient autonomy (Robertson 1996). However, for reasons that I discuss further in Chapter 8, nurses tend to see liberty in apolitical terms, as the autonomy of the private individual rather than the liberty of the citizen.

Arguably nursing's emphasis on care is by contrast geared to supporting the patient in the citizen. Care is not a principle that sits well with the moral position of the citizen, and the relation of citizen to citizen, as it implies an individualised commitment which runs counter to the even-handedness of the citizen role. But it is clearly an important principle in relation to the patient, and to the nurse-patient relationship. An issue arises here about rationality, however. The assumption that the citizen will behave rationally is clearly often wrong. Frequently citizens do nothing of the sort. Often that does not matter greatly. But if the citizen-as-patient makes unwise and irrational decisions about agreeing to treatment, this may be a matter of life and death. So, the citizen needs to be sustained in her or his rationality in a situation where that rationality is particularly difficult to sustain. The nurse's role in this is clearly crucial, through supporting the patient in rational decision-making and seeking to minimise the kind of stresses that undermine rationality.

So far I have considered this in the context of citizens rights that belong in the liberal framework. The social democrat framework has a more extensive view of social rights – those rights which involve the provision of specific goods to the citizen by the state or public bodies. In a state-provided health service health care, including nursing care, must fall within the meaning of the citizen's social rights. In a limited sense the nurse is upholding that right simply by providing nursing care, but to be truly a guardian of citizen rights in that context the nurse should be going further to ensure that the patient is receiving his or her full entitlement of care and treatment. Writers on nursing ethics such as S. Edwards (1996) give some emphasis to the issue of justice, and to the nurse's role in seeking to ensure a just distribution of resources to patients, and a fair availability of care in accordance with citizen rights. It can also be included in the concept of patient advocacy. The code of professional conduct can be interpreted as enjoining the same commitment, although this is more ambiguous. The process of advocating for patients social right to a particular resource is clearly rather different from the process of advocating for patients civil right to autonomy and given the position of nurses in the care system, and their historic lack of involvement in resource allocation, perhaps more difficult.

The nurse and the duties of the citizen

A nursing commitment to support and sustain the citizenship and citizen-rights of patients seems to fit well with nursing ethics and the nurse's role in modern health care. However, we need to ask also whether a case can be made for nurses helping patients to fulfil their duties as citizens. *The NHS Guide* (Department of Health 2000) identifies a set of expectations upon the patient/citizen that stand alongside their rights to care. These include an expectation of reasonable behaviour in relation to health care professionals and the NHS, and also an expectation of healthy living. So this is now part of public discourse in the NHS. But that does not necessarily mean that it becomes part of the nurse's role to reinforce these expectations. Should nurses concern themselves with the degree to which their patients are respecting the liberty of others, for instance, or dealing honestly with others? Most patients are not in a position to seriously threaten the liberty, or safety, of others. Some of those who do behave in a threatening way do so because they are mentally ill or intoxicated and unable to rationally consider their rights and duties. With others (for instance in busy casualty wards) threatening behaviour often constitutes a risk to other patients, and the nurse's duty to provide care for patients would prompt them to intervene in any case in that situation, even if they had no commitment to reminding the recalcitrant patient of his citizen duty. Where those who are suffering from the threatening patient's behaviour are not themselves patients, it is hard to find instances where it makes sense to involve the nurse in reinforcing the patient's duty as a citizen. I referred above to the contractual element in the nurse-citizen relationship, and the importance of the code of professional conduct as an expression of professional commitment. A close reading of the code offers nothing that could provide a basis for arguing that nurses are committed to doing this.

I mentioned above the nurse's role in supporting the patient's welfare rights. Traditionally nurses have not engaged with the opposite role, that of guardian of resources. But if we take welfare rights to be accompanied by a duty to make appropriate use of welfare resources, and not to use them dishonestly or otherwise inappropriately to the detriment of needy fellow citizens, then performance of such a duty becomes the legitimate business of those professionals whose job it is to provide health care in accordance with patients' rights and needs. That is not to say that they have the job also of monitoring the behaviour of patients in this respect and pointing out to them if they seem to be in breach of this duty. But they are in an exceptionally advantageous position to do this. In practice nurses and other health care professionals do feel able on occasions to point out to patients that their prodigal use of health care resources are depriving others of what they need. But that does not mean that this would be accepted as part of their formal role. Again, if we take the contractual relationship between nurse and patient defined in the code of professional conduct as our reference point, there is no moral basis for such a role.

However, a different view can be taken of this if we move away from the liberal and social democratic frameworks and take a civic republican view of the citizen's role as patient. A contractual view of the nurse's role fits well with the liberal perspective in that it assumes no obligations exist other than those specifically entered into. By contrast the civic republican view would be that obligations are built into the citizen role and that nurses are citizens with specific abilities and opportunities to engage with other citizens in relation to their civic duty. Sorrell (2001) takes up this issue in relation to medicine, and argues that the citizen role of patients and professionals does involve obligations on the part of the patient as well as on the professional, and particularly that the patient has duties to the professional as well as vice versa. The same arguments can be readily extended to nursing. In particular, Sorrell's argument that the vulnerability of patients does not absolve them from duties, is helpful in this context. However, as ever, the difficulty is to agree on precisely what the duties are. As Mouffe (1993) points out Civic Republicanism requires a degree of moral consensus that seems to be receding in late modern societies. The civic role of nurse-as-citizen, is according to Nelson (2001) very much part of the history of nursing in the early twentieth century, despite having retreated somewhat from nursing discourse in recent decades. I consider in Chapter 8 whether a more active political engagement makes sense for nursing in the present situation, where consensus on civic and citizen obligations is lacking.

Family relationships

There are other roles than that of the citizen, in which nurses will interact with patients. In day-to-day living, and in matters of health care and treatment, probably the most important in affecting the relationship between nurse and patient are family roles. The expectations that belong to the role of citizen are clearly different, and differently based, from those that belong to the role of spouse, parent or offspring. In family relationships we expect a degree of altruism, and in some family relationships a high degree, shading into self-sacrifice in some situations. We expect that family relationships will often not be characterised by rationality any more than they are by self-interest, and we tend to accept a degree of irrational behaviour as inevitable even if this can be seen to be counter-productive. A good example of this is 'stranger danger' panic among parents of young children, which bears no proportional relationships to actual risk. We may need also to accept that different moral principles apply to at least some family relationships. That people favour their own relatives against others in distributing their goods, attention and concern is something that denies the equal worth of all persons, and clearly goes against the kind of even-handed morality that seems to apply to citizenship. But it is something that, far from being inappropriate in family life, seems to be an inevitable part thereof, and for most people an appropriate part. All this raises the question of what moral principles should be applied to family relationships.

In addressing this problem McConaghy and Cottone (1998) make a useful distinction between the view of family relationships as driven by 'natural' processes which they term 'exogenic', and the view of the same processes that accommodates individual responsibility and autonomy, a view they term 'endogenic'. They argue that to understand and work effectively with families (they write as family therapists) the endogenic view needs to be included in the professional's perspective and practice. Their argument is both a theoretical and a practical one in terms of engaging effectively with families. If individual responsibility (and the moral implications of this) are inescapable even at this deepest level of family dynamics, we can reasonably argue that family relationships are every bit as much in need of a clear moral perspective as are citizen-to-citizen relationships.

But what kind of moral perspective can we apply to the family? We could apply the same principles to family roles as we applied to the role of citizen. We could look for a utilitarian justification for family loyalty, and such a justification is arguable to a degree. There are general benefits from the family as an institution that might maximise happiness. A utilitarian might argue this, although the lack of a clear alternative with which to make a comparison creates difficulties. If we cannot realistically envisage replacing family relationships with something else, the argument that families offer the best option for well-being becomes trivial, as it is the only option. If we look at the details of family behaviour – the degree to which and the ways in which family members favour one another and the demands they make on one another – we might also find utilitarian justifications for many actions performed in that context. But we are equally likely to conclude that much family-centred behaviour does not maximise well-being and cannot be justified in that way. Nor does Kantian morality solve any problems in this area. Its emphasis on universal respect for persons does not fit with the specificity of family relationships. The only element that might fit with some family relationships is the injunction to keep promises, one of the well-known applications of Kant's categorical imperative. This could be applied to spouse relationships, where it may provide a degree of structure to the complex business of balancing the needs and aspirations of couples as they develop and change. It is hard to see how other kinds of family relationship could be brought into this kind of framework, however, as promises play little or no part in underpinning them.

The concept of care, which forms an important component of nursing ethics, seems to be a potentially useful concept also for family ethics. It would be feasible (although not always easy) to distinguish between actions characterised by care for another person in the family, and those that are motivated by other factors. It would be feasible to accept a variation in the degree of care appropriate in different kinds of family relationship. The focus on care allows the non-rational element in behaviour to be accommodated, but at the same time it requires a degree of commitment to fulfil the requirements of a care-based family morality, in that care does not involve simply the expression of a caring impulse, but also a commitment to empathy with the other person.

There is evidence that the behaviour of people in family relationships is strongly affected by moral principles, in particular the principle of duty, and that this, more than anything else, makes family relationships different from other relationships. Finch and Mason (Finch 1989; Finch and Mason 1993) in their study identified a distinct set of moral precepts, centring round duty, in the family behaviour of their subjects. However, these precepts were largely implicit rather than explicit in the thinking of her subjects, and their observance was modified by considerations of rational self-interest. Barlow and Duncan (2000) similarly argue that family behaviour is both moral and rational, though the morality arises from a process of negotiation which is contingent on social norms rather than based on absolute principles.

However, family practice seems to be changing. There is still a strong conception of parental duty, and a weakening conception of parental rights, in our legal system, which to some degree reflects the ethics of the community and to some extent seeks to influence these (see, for instance, Harding 1994). There is a general acceptance that parents have a duty to provide care for their children, and that children have a right to this. The obverse of this, children's duties and parents rights, are both seen as problematic in contemporary society. There is a great deal of variation in people's views as to what if any rights people have to the care or attention of their offspring or of other relatives; or conversely of what duties if any people owe to their parents, or other relatives. Social expectations of care of spouse by spouse are still considerably affected by gender. In terms of care provided by parents for children it seems to make sense to have a family morality based around care because there seems a sufficient degree of consensus to sustain this. However, other family relationships do not enjoy anything like the same degree of consensus. There is evidence from Davies (2000) that traditional views of family obligation for care for elderly parents and other dependent relatives are in sharp retreat As part of the process of individualisation in western culture it seems that the concept of family duty is losing its hold outside of the parent-child dyad.

The nurse and family relationships

For many patients their family roles are far more important in their own scale of priorities than their role as citizen. This will particularly be the case when they are receiving health care. So nurses are likely to encounter these roles in an especially overt way. Certain areas of practice such as health visiting are clearly engaged with supporting the right of children to care by their parents, and in supporting parents in performing the duty of caring for their children. This is clearly in accordance with the expressed values of nursing, and it does not involve an explicit promotion of parental duty. Some observers, for instance J. Edwards (1996), suggest that the idea of parental duty is *implicit* in health visitors' accounts of their work, and this may be a potent sub-text, but it does not have the legitimacy to be part of any explicit contract between professional and client. In respect of parents, the health visitor's balance between support and authority has always veered toward support, and the more authoritarian role tends to be taken by other professionals, particularly social workers who, paradoxically, seem according to Dalley (1993) more ideologically opposed to the idea of family duty.

In other aspects of family life the picture is even less clear. Who has a duty of care toward whom within the family is a matter so lacking in consensus that it is very difficult to suggest any professional role in respect of these. Clearly nurses and doctors are both on occasion drawn into exhorting relatives to provide care in order to relieve the pressure on inadequate health or social care resources. This is probably a pragmatic response on many occasions, but that is not to deny that professionals may choose to confront relatives on principle. Dalley found evidence that some nurses do subscribe to a view that relatives have a duty to care for their elderly and infirm. Whether the promotion of that principle to relatives and patients is a valid professional role is much more doubtful, however. In the absence of a social consensus on this, and in the absence of a clear commitment in the code of conduct of the profession there seems no secure basis for this.

Healthy living

One major area remains to be considered in respect of the nurse's relationship with the patient as citizen, and because of its importance I propose to deal with it separately and at some length. This concerns the individual's influence on their own health, which can be related to the use they make of the NHS. We know that the treatment of smoking-related diseases accounts for a substantial element of the NHS budget every year, and that most of this is preventable through changes in the behaviour of citizens. A similar argument applies to several other areas of health care, to varying degrees. Obesity is an increasing threat to health, and again much of this is preventable on the basis of the freely chosen behaviour of citizens. In this connection we may ask whether citizens have a duty to the state and their fellow citizens to guard their health and thereby show due regard for the fact that the price of their self-destructive behaviour would be paid by their fellow citizens. The expectations upon the patient presented in *The NHS Guide* (Department of Health 2000) include an expectation to live a healthy life-style. These expectations are on the face of it modest and commonsensical, but it is possible to see them as part of a shift in government thinking toward a greater reciprocity of duties and rights between citizen and state, a shift identified in other contexts by Lund (1999) and by Lister (1998). It may be that we can see civic republican ideas creeping into government thinking. If healthy living is being represented as a citizen duty, we must in due course ask what the nurse's role is in relation to that duty.

Arguments can be identified against the idea of a duty of reasonable self-care. One such argument would be that it is a denial of individual autonomy to impose on people an obligation to restrict their activities when these are harmless to all except themselves. A rather different argument would be that it is unreasonable to impose a duty on people to resist what may be overwhelming cultural pressure to do dangerous and self-destructive things like drink too much alcohol, overeat and have unsafe sex; and it would be even more unreasonable to withhold health care, or otherwise penalise people, for doing what their free will, or their culture, legitimately prompt (Persaud 1995).

Against this we could argue that the existence of a moral duty (as opposed to a legal duty) does not entail enforcement. The Kantian idea of duty as an inner moral compass does not entail any notion that people should be forced to do their moral duty. This would be a denial of the element of choice that is essential to the Kantian idea of ethics, as it is to the idea of the citizen. That is not to say that wrongful acts cannot be punished by the appropriate authorities, but many duty-bound actions in Kant's scheme, such as promise-keeping, are only enforced legally in certain specific situations. Usually promises are broken with legal impunity. So a duty to guard one's health need not be legally enforceable, or enforceable in any other way, to be seen as a moral duty to one's fellow citizens. It certainly need not involve withholding health care resources from self-damaging patients, as it does not follow from failing in a duty of self-care, that one's right to health care is negated. In response to the argument from cultural pressure, we can argue that cultural pressures exist to do many things that are in breach of identifiable duties – to lie, to break promises, to evade taxes – but that we can still clearly distinguish between behaviour that is a social norm in a particular society and behaviour that is regarded as morally right in that society. In all such areas the existence of morality rests upon the principle that in significant respects most people have enough choice to be ascribed some responsibility for their actions.

Perhaps the main argument in favour of recognising a duty to guard one's health rests on the reciprocity of taxpayer and patient. Taxes must be paid on the implicit agreement that the money will be used effectively to achieve particular shared ends, including better health. If a patient negates treatment that he is receiving, by continuing to smoke, he is preventing that money from being spent to good effect. If a patient knowingly damages his health and requires health resources to be spent on him relatively ineffectively, he is 'wasting' his neighbour's taxes just as if he continues to smoke during or after treatment. The effects of smoking, excessive drinking and obesity, are less likely to trigger curable diseases that cost money to cure, than they are to bring on or hasten incurable chronic or life-threatening diseases where the expenditure of health care resources is relatively wasteful in relation to health gain. The patient in this situation also renders his neighbour's taxes relatively ineffective, and so negates to some degree the benefits of paying those taxes for the rest of the community. If the government has a duty to use taxes for the greatest possible benefit of the community, then each citizen arguably has a duty to allow that to happen. To say this is not to suggest that treatment should be withheld from the self-destructive patient. My argument for a duty to guard one's health in fact depends on a principle that, once it is damaged, the patient has the same right to treatment as the patient whose conditions not a result of chosen behaviour.

If we accept for the moment that there is a duty on the citizen to guard her or his own health, what does this imply for the nurse's situation? Does it mean that nurses have a role in encouraging patients to fulfil their duty to their fellow citizens and guard their own health? Clearly nurses have an important health promotion role that involves encouraging patients to guard their health in any case. But whatever skills and resources are used to achieve this can be adequately justified by the resultant benefit to the patient and the community, in accordance with professional principles and the terms of the code of professional conduct. This is quite different from encouraging patients to fulfil a duty to the rest of the community and the state, and we need to ask whether the latter is any part of the nurse's professional role. The answer, probably, is no. If we look at those documents and statements that express to the community the professional commitment of nursing, it does not include the promotion of any principles of public morality, and the kind of social solidarity that is implicit in the code of conduct does not stretch to this social obligation. This is an important point because it says something about the degree of pressure that is legitimate to use on smokers, drinkers and other self-damaging citizens. Likewise we have to conclude that there is nothing in the nurse's contract with the community or the state that requires working for the benefit of the taxpayer. The professional role of the nurse is focused primarily on the health and care of the individual, and to a lesser degree that of the community. Other beneficiaries and other benefits are secondary.

Exploring the same issue from a utilitarian perspective it is interesting to consider in general how far we should go in exerting pressure on people to live healthy lives, without the balance-sheet of gain and loss of well-being going against us. There is clearly a point at which other losses, for instance of autonomy, would detract from well-being, if we applied too much pressure on people to live healthy lives. Incentives can shade into threats, persuasion into manipulation, and health gain can be countered by losses in other goods that also contribute to well-being. However, it is particularly difficult to establish at what point that balance is reached, because, I would suggest, this is one of the areas where lack of social consensus makes it very difficult to agree on the relative benefits of health and other goods. The enjoyment of risky sports can be set against health. The enjoyment of unhealthy indulgences such as tobacco, alcohol, other recreational drugs, and unsafe sex can likewise be seen as an authentic source of well-being. The motor car provides an enormous range of enriching opportunities, as well as a threat to health. And many industrial processes which damage the environment and damage health, also contribute to the quality and enjoyment of life on a material level. Our patterns of consumption which are often unhealthy, are essential for the sustaining of a post-industrial economy, and of the standard of living that that provides. All are sources of happiness, and some are no doubt sources of wisdom and beauty. The relative balance in terms of the well-being afforded by all these activities, as against that of good health, is likely to vary between individuals, between communities, between cultures and between age-groups. On a deeper level it is also argued by writers such as O'Brien (1995) that health promotion can provide a means of colonisation of culture and society by state and other bodies with a controlling, manipulative agenda. Vague, ever-broadening definitions of health and well-being facilitate this process. In this argument freedom itself is potentially in conflict with the promotion of health.

This seems to leave nurses without a firm moral basis to judge the vigour of their advocacy of healthy living. However, it is one of the fundamental themes of this book that nurses must operate in a society where consensus on the value of what they do is lacking. They cannot look to the rest of society for a clear message as to what they should do. I argued in Chapter 1 that health is a good which, although not in itself a moral good like justice, provides a moral basis for acting to promote it, as do other goods such as wisdom, beauty and happiness. I would argue on that basis that the promotion of health is justifiable in its own right, as is promotion of the other goods I have mentioned. There is a strong argument for ensuring, in the absence of shared priorities, that a range of goods is promoted, providing choice and balance. Where we cannot agree what is good, we need to be able to draw on a variety of options. It is appropriate therefore for each of those goods to be promoted with conviction by responsible groups, so that they remain well embedded in the discourse of that society. Nursing has a considerable contribution to make to the process of ensuring that health stays strongly present in the value repertoire of our society and the cultures that constitute it. The promotion of health on an individual and collective level can be seen as part of this enterprise. Where health priorities conflict with other priorities based on other goods, we cannot always argue health should prevail, but we can argue that it should have honest and responsible advocacy. The nursing profession is probably the most effective group fulfilling that role. The relative openness of the nursing view of health is suited to the situation of uncertainty. And the element of distance in the relationship between the nursing profession and the state means that the role of nursing in promoting health can be to some degree independent of immediate government agendas.

Conclusion

The rights and duties of the citizen are in many respects unclear and problematic, as are the moral status of the family and the role of the individual within it. These uncertainties apply to many aspects of individual behaviour and relationships, and they apply in particular to health-related behaviour. All this makes the relationship of the nurse to the citizen very unclear, as nurses are deprived of a framework of agreed principles on which to ground their actions.

5 Nursing and organisations

Introduction

This chapter considers the role and functions of organisations in health and social care, and reflects on their duties and relationships in relation to the citizen, the state and one another. A similar analysis is undertaken in relation to teams, with a particular focus on interprofessional and inter-organisational teams. The position of the nursing profession and of the individual nurse in this context constitutes a continuing theme throughout the chapter.

Why organisations matter

The nurse's relationship to the state, and to the patient, is mediated by a variety of organisations – strategic health authorities, NHS trusts, primary care trusts and elected local authorities. Most nurses are employees of organisations and their dealings with patients are undertaken in the role of employee as well as in the role of professional. And although most nurses are employees of the state health care system, the state has conferred a good deal of corporate autonomy on the bodies that actually deliver health care and employ nurses. So these organisations need to be considered in their own right in the nurse's moral and political landscape. As the bodies charged with the duty of delivering health care, their policies and practices have a major impact on the quality of care received by patients. The nurse's professional duty to the patient – among other things, to act always for the patient's benefit – may on occasions come into conflict with the practices of the trust or PCT. Those practices may not always benefit the patient, and the nurse may feel duty-bound to respond to this, and to consider how she should behave toward the organisation, both as an employee and as a professional. In this, her judgement of the ethics of her position and of the organisation's position becomes important.

Corporate ethics

I have referred to organisations having duties, and in that respect my language implies an equation of organisational behaviour with individual behaviour. But we must consider the ethics of organisational actions in more depth. When we say 'the trust did this' or 'the PCT decided that' does that imply that an organisation can in these respects behave like a person, that it is an agent, with the power to make decisions and take actions? Or are we simply using a form of shorthand where the term 'trust' or 'PCT' works as an impersonal stand-in for one or more human beings to whom we are really referring? We could be referring to the chief executive, the board, specific managers at any level, depending on the context. If it is impossible for organisations to 'do things' as human beings do, then it must be that we are referring implicitly to collections of individuals. If organisations can 'do things' then we can ascribe actions and decisions to them.

This issue is a matter of debate, particularly in business ethics, and a good deal seems to depend on what we read into the idea of agency and responsibility. In terms of agency, organisations cannot literally act as humans can because they are not corporeal beings with bodies that can respond to volition, suggests Velasquez (1983). And in terms of moral status and responsibility, it makes no sense to ascribe moral qualities to the motives of organisations, as we could to a human. On the other hand as French (1979) argues, there are situations where the action of an organisation is not reducible to the actions of any individual, and there seems no alternative but to ascribe it to the organisation.

That is not to say that organisations are 'person-like' in other ways. If we use a Kantian definition of 'person', organisations clearly do not qualify because they are not ends in themselves. Unlike persons whose existence is self-justifying in the Kantian framework, organisations must exist for a purpose, because they only come into existence through the purposeful behaviour of persons. So a company is set up for the purpose of making money for its shareholders or owner. These are the people who legitimise the company's existence and purpose, and it is to them that it is ultimately accountable. They provide the company's 'constituency' (Wilmot 1997). A NHS trust is set up by the government with the purpose of delivering a particular kind of health care to a particular population. So central government is the trust's constituency. It legitimises the existence and purpose of the trust, and it is the government to which the trust is accountable. It provides it with its 'ends'. For this reason organisations must always be morally secondary to persons.

However, the fact that organisations exist for a purpose is as important as the way they behave, at least for their employees and for others who need to decide how to respond to that behaviour. An organisation that exists to make money for its shareholders or owner exists for a purpose that is essentially amoral. It is neither morally good nor morally bad and can be seen as part of a process through which people rationally pursue their self-interest. The purpose of a NHS trust – to provide health care – is by contrast seeking to provide a service to a population which is geared to optimising a particular good for that population. This places it in a rather different category from the commercial enterprise. The trust is seeking to treat the recipients of its service as ends, and it is seeking to distribute a good conducive to well-being as widely as it is able. In that sense it is 'doing the right thing', both in Kantian and in utilitarian terms. The commercial company is likely to be treating its customers to a greater degree as means to its own end, and its own end is to make money for its own constituency. The moral difference between the two is considerable (Wilmot 2000). If we are to make choices based on promoting what is morally good, the trust should be favoured over the company. Where a trust is seen by its employees as acting wrongly or irresponsibly, the judgement as to the right response may be rather different as a result of this. A response that is damaging to the organisation, particularly where that damage might prevent it from fulfilling its purpose, may be less appropriate where the organisation exists for a purpose that is morally good. For the nurse, the moral good built into the purpose of the trust is doubly compelling because it relates to the particular goods that the nursing profession primarily espouses – health and care. The issue of nurses acting against their employers for professional reasons is explored further in Chapter 10.

At the beginning of the chapter I said that most nurses in the UK are employed within the system of state health care. However, a significant minority of the profession are located in the private and voluntary sectors, working for private providers of care such as private nursing homes and private hospitals, or for voluntary organisations in various capacities. We need to consider therefore what moral considerations apply to such organisations. With regard to the private sector I suggested earlier that a commercial company exists first to make a profit for its shareholders or owner. They are the company's constituency, the people who legitimise the existence of the company and give it its purpose, and generally that is the purpose they give it. A company's management may choose to embrace a duty to customers, to employees, even to the community at large. But that is something they can equally 'unchoose' if it suits them, unless the requirement is enforced by law. The duty to shareholders or owner is not a matter of choice. The shareholders or owner may choose to give priority to the standard of care provided in their nursing homes, as against the profits they derive from it. But that is their choice, and they are equally free to give priority to their own profit at the expense of patient care (assuming they are staying within legal regulation). There is nothing built into the purpose or mandate of such an organisation, as there is to that of the NHS trust, giving first priority to its provision of health care.

This aspect of the situation is important as the private sector is drawn increasingly into providing services for the NHS through recent government initiatives. In this context I would argue that the private health care provider does not acquire a new constituency as a result of providing NHS services. The relationships between the NHS and the private provider are contractual, as the NHS is in effect buying the services of the private provider. The NHS will be in the role of customer, and the level of quality which the private provider chooses to commit themselves to (and adhere to) will be ultimately for them a matter of maximising profit, as with any other transaction.

This means that the position of the nurse working in the private sector differs significantly from that of the state sector nurse. In the state sector the nurse can suppose that there is a degree of common purpose between herself as a professional, and the organisation she works for. In the private sector she cannot have this expectation. In the state sector where trust management are failing to provide adequate care in a way that is affecting the nurse's ability to practice appropriately, she can argue that management are failing to pursue their own purpose and acting against the trusts interests as well as those of the patient. In the private sector she cannot argue this. However, it is not clear that in practice this makes much difference, or that the private sector is in any general sense a worse provider than the state sector. Both are subject to financial constraints, though of different kinds, and both kinds of management will doubtless argue (sometimes justifiably) that this forces them to provide worse care than they would wish. There may be a difference in the kind of obligations that the nurse might accept toward her employer on the basis of common moral goals.

The position of the nurse in the voluntary sector is rather different. Voluntary bodies are essentially answerable to their members, as companies are answerable to their shareholders. The difference is that members of voluntary bodies are not seeking a dividend, and are usually involved because of a commitment to improving the position of a particular patient/client population. So for the nurse working in that setting the conflict between commitment to patient care and accountability to membership is not likely to be a problem, as members' and patients' interests are more likely to coincide (they may in many cases be the same people). However, dilemmas of a different sort may arise. Voluntary bodies have been increasingly drawn into contractual relationships with the NHS as service providers in recent years, but they remain in many cases also campaigning organisations, working to promote the well-being of particular groups. This produces some confusion of aims, and, Stalker *et al.* (1999) argue, confusion of values and ideology. However, it remains the case that they are under no obligation to be even-handed between different patient groups as are NHS bodies. Often voluntary bodies exist to pursue the claims of a particular group. Also they may be committed to advocating the virtues of particularly treatments or methods of care, for political rather than scientific or professional reasons. This may present particular problems for the nurse who is professionally committed to evidence-based practice and who may therefore identify a conflict between her role as employee, supporting her employer's methods, and her role as professional, subjecting those same methods to critical appraisal.

Organisations delivering health and social care

The NHS consists of a complex network of organisations with varying degrees of autonomy. The health care system as a whole includes an even wider and more diverse range of organisations (since the private and voluntary sectors must be included) and if we include social care the range becomes wider still. We need to consider the relationships that connect these organisations to co-ordinate their activities and deliver a national system of health care. In ethical and political terms the key bond is that of accountability. So first, we must ask what accountability exists between health authorities and trusts and their environment. Crucially, as Hutton (2000) points out, there is no direct formal relationship of accountability between any of these bodies and the public. They are not elected, so the electorate cannot hold them accountable. Their accountability is upward, to bodies higher in the hierarchy of organisations, and to the secretary of state. Democratic accountability is only expressed in a circuitous fashion, through the fact that the secretary of state is formally accountable to parliament. In practice health authorities and trusts have sought to communicate with the populations they serve, particularly to seek their views and explain their policies and practices (e.g. Hope *et al.* 1998). But there is no formal machinery whereby the local population can hold one of these bodies democratically accountable.

This can be contrasted with local authorities, which are equivalent in many ways to health providers in their function, but which have a clear relationship of democratic accountability through the fact that their governing bodies are elected. As Wilson and Game (1998) make clear, though local authorities are subordinate to central government, that relationship is balanced (and often complicated) by their accountability to the local electorate. This contrast highlights the democratic deficit in the NHS, which is paradoxically exposed even further by the use of democratic and participatory rhetoric by government in relation to health as, for instance, in Saving Lives (Department of Health 1999) and by attempts to introduce local representation into primary care through the inclusion of lay representatives on PCT boards. The limited nature of such representation, when set against the aforementioned rhetoric, emphasises rather than disguises the democratic deficit. As Hogg and Williamson (2001) point out, lay representatives on health bodies arrive with widely differing agendas, and in some cases they will be predisposed to support those groups and individuals who are in a dominant position. Lay representatives with a more oppositional agenda are likely to find themselves in a very small minority.

The kind of relationships that exist between organisations within health and social care is a vital part of the overall context of nursing. The reforms of 1990 sought to create an internal market in which health authorities and fundholding GPs purchased services for their populations and patients from NHS trusts. The buyer/seller distinction was intended to create incentives for services to become both more efficient and of higher quality. Because the NHS was never a true market, and the market mechanism (essentially competition) was allowed only very limited play, the desired effect on efficiency was not achieved. However, other effects did follow. It is clear as Hunter (1997) points out that the internal market profoundly changed the relationships between different components of the NHS in the direction of greater conflict of interest, and a diminished sense of common purpose. Conflict certainly existed in the pre-1990 NHS, between hospitals, between professional groups and between authorities. In Klein's (1995) account of the 1948–90 period there is certainly no lack of such conflict. However, in Hunter's view there was also a general understanding that people in the NHS were working roughly toward the same ends, and that mistrust and conflict, while unavoidable to a degree, were problems to be managed and minimised. After 1990 the internal market changed these relationships by institutionalising conflicts of interest. The shared sense of common purpose receded in the face of increased mistrust between buyers and sellers, and among potentially competing sellers.

New Labour's policies after 1997 sought to reverse this trend by laying upon the component organisations of the NHS a duty of co-operation with one another, and with other bodies (Department of Health 1997). Over the next few years it may be that this will change the atmosphere and the kind of dealings which NHS organisations engage in with one another. However, it is not clear that this will necessarily lead to a return to the situation before 1990. The likelihood is that the post-1999 NHS will still be a relatively conflictual place. First, old habits die hard, as Baker (2000) points out. Many key personnel learned their skills in the early to mid 1990s when competitiveness was at a premium. Second, the potential for conflict increases with the number of players. The number of distinct organisations controlling substantial resources has been greatly increased by the creation of primary care groups and primary care trusts. Also the internal structures of these bodies may contribute to the problem. According to Meads and Ashcroft (2000), they have emerged in many cases as very loose, with highly permeable boundaries. They characterise these bodies as 'virtual organisations', with highly devolved structures. They also use the concept of 'stakeholder organisations' to describe PCTs, based on the close involvement of representatives of other bodies in governing them. Though this structure is in part intended to avoid conflict, there is certainly the potential for the opposite effect. The other relationship which can never be conflict-free is that between commissioner and provider. Even though co-operation is enjoined, the interests of commissioner and provider can never entirely coincide. Finally, the sheer complexity of co-ordinating a system involving numerous distinct organisations and systems will lead to misunderstandings, miscommunications and mistakes that will themselves create tensions and conflict within and between organisations.

The statutory duty of co-operation also covers co-operation with bodies outside of the NHS such as local authorities. It will be interesting to see how that duty works out in practice. There is some evidence from Hiscock and Pearson (1999) that health bodies and social service agencies and personnel became more distant and distrustful of one another as a result of their experiences in the internal market. This would suggest there is distance to make up. But Hudson (2000), reporting on post-1998 collaboration within the nascent PCGs, is more optimistic that co-operation at the 'stakeholder' level now has the prospect of success. Hudson focuses on the managerial level of collaboration. But there are other levels where difficulties may still arise in terms of differing constituencies and conflicting accountability. Major policy developments such as the introduction of the internal market (Department of Health 1989), and the *NHS Plan* (Department of Health 2000) have tended to assume a superficial homogeneity among public bodies, putting local authorities alongside appointed bodies such as health authorities, trusts and PCTs in a somewhat undifferentiated manner. But the truth is, as Loughlin (1996) points out, that local authorities have much deeper and more autonomous constitutional roots than health care bodies, and as elected bodies they have a relationship of both accountability and duty to their local electorate. Loughlin argues that this has a legal expression in the fiduciary relationship between local authority and its council taxpayers, laying a duty of trust on the local authority, to spend its resources fairly and to the benefit of its taxpayers.

This duty exists independently of local authority obligations to central government, which is the basis of their duty of co-operation with health bodies. And it is quite possible that these duties will conflict. Already the basis for such a conflict exists in the Wyre Forest district of the West Midlands where the local population expressed its anger at health authority policy by making a protest vote (and electing protest candidates) in local authority elections (Gulland 2001). Collaboration could become very complicated if this were to happen more widely. Organisations will need to decide how far they are willing to compromise on their own conception of their mandate, their purpose, and therefore their interests, in order to comply with the duty of co-operation.

The situation described above throws up several challenges for nurses. Nurses unlike, for instance, social workers, are not on the whole strongly organisation-conscious. A situation where organisations are developing in primary care into somewhat fluid, intertwined, even 'virtual' forms may seem promising for a profession impatient with procedures and bureaucracy. However, the complexity and unpredictability of the situation emerging may present more difficulties for those who are less oriented toward organisational issues. For nurses who have looked to provider organisations to offer a reliable, stable, taken-for-granted structure within which they can continue to provide patient care, the emerging situation will be challenging. The other potential challenge to nurses arises from conflicts that might emerge in this context, as different organisations are required to combine, and even merge, their functions. One setting where the potential conflicts of interest between local authorities and NHS organisations described above may manifest is the care trust, a new body providing combined health and social care and jointly run by health bodies and local authorities. Care trusts are already being suspected by some social work commentators of being, at least potentially, an instrument for subordinating social services to the NHS (Bywaters and McLeod 2001) and comments by individual social workers on this issue suggest there may be something of an ideological rearguard action in prospect (Gibb and Pryde 2001). Again, nurses are likely to be the main face-to-face protagonists with social workers in this. The culture of nursing is strongly focused toward consensus and away from overt ideological conflict, so this situation will also be a challenge.

Team responsibility

Although corporate identity may lie with the trust or PCT, the reality of shared decision-making and responsibility is more directly experienced at the team level. Much direct service delivery is organised around teams, and it is through the team that the individual nurse will most frequently experience the organisation. This means that the individual's moral relationship with the organisation consists of three relationships – the relationship of the individual to the organisation as a whole; the relationship of the individual to the team; and the relationship of the team to the organisation. The first of these three has already been considered to some degree, so the other two need some consideration.

Teams are not corporate bodies. Although some small organisations (usually voluntary or private) consist of one team, this is unusual in the NHS. Usually teams are groupings of varying degrees of stability, which are part of the internal structure of a corporate organisation. This means that teams have a rather different moral status from organisations. Whereas we can talk of a decision by the trust, which is actually a decision by a small body of managers or a single chief executive representing the trust, we cannot normally talk about a team decision unless the team members are directly involved in making the decision. If the team leader makes the decision on her own, then we would say that it is a decision of the team leader, not of the team. We would only refer to a team decision if all team members have the opportunity to be involved in it. This difference demonstrates the fact that the operation of the team *as* a team generally depends on the involvement of all team members. In this sense team responsibility – the responsibility of the team for actions taken by it – falls into a different category form the responsibly of organisations. French (1984) argues that whereas organisations with formal decisions structures could be said to have corporate responsibility – responsibly which belongs entirely to the collectivity and does not necessarily imply any individual responsibility on the part of any individual member of that collectivity – less formal groupings may be ascribed aggregate responsibility, wherein responsibility for the actions of the collectivity is in fact reducible to the responsibility of every individual in that collectivity for those actions. This seems to come nearer to the team situation.

Where a team is functioning as a decision-making collectivity, the distribution of responsibility for its service delivery still raises some problems. Ovretveit (1993) has identified three quite distinct kinds of team leadership, with very different implications in terms of responsibility. Using his terminology, where the team is led by a 'chairperson' whose function is mainly to facilitate team decision-making, responsibility for team actions need not fall disproportionately on that individual. Where the team has fair decision-making procedures, and the chairperson facilitates these appropriately, responsibility will be distributed equally throughout the team. By contrast, where a leader in the 'team manager' role, leads the team with full managerial accountability for the work of all team members, that leader must carry a disproportionate moral responsibility for team actions, simply as a result of the power vested in that role. Ovretveit's intermediate position, the 'co-ordinator', involves some administrative and co-ordinating responsibility that would in some situations lead that individual to carry disproportionate responsibility for team functioning, but not necessarily for team decisions.

We then encounter questions of collective and individual commitment to team decisions. There are a number of reasons why an individual team member may not have personally agreed to a particular decision, but might still be seen as sharing responsibility for it. If the team has a decision-making procedure that allows for the decisions to be made without all members present, and that procedure has the agreement of all team members, then all members can be seen as party to decisions falling within that agreement. This may include the absence of one or two members from meetings, and the delegation of particular decisions to part of the team. The prior agreement of all team members to those procedures, and to the kind of decisions that fall within those procedures, would seem to constitute a sufficiently promise-like contract to provide a secure moral basis for such an arrangement.

However, social realities sometimes undermine rational frameworks. In small-group situations it is not difficult for individuals to become intimidated and disabled by patterns of communication. Particular ways of presenting information or opinions, while not overtly dishonest, can be confusing and disempowering. Particular kinds of terminology can produce anxiety and loss of confidence. Personal advantages of education, skill or confidence can be used in ways that marginalise other members. The inequalities of power and influence that such patterns produce are known to have a depressive effect on group functioning, other things being equal (Johnson and Johnson 1987; van Dyne and Saavedra 1996).

All these considerations are relevant to the position of nurses in the team context. The team is the forum where the nursing agenda on health can be developed in the greatest depth and detail, and where the nursing profession can be most comprehensively involved. The team is the place where the nature and value of health can be most effectively reviewed and clarified, and through this medium the organisation can be influenced also. Nurses often constitute the majority, or the biggest single element, in teams within the NHS, this being an unsurprising consequence of their numerical preponderance in the workforce. However, this does not mean that they are accustomed to dominating the typical NHS team in terms of power. The unequal relationship that has existed between the medical and nursing professions often manifests itself in the team context (Dombeck 1997). If the nursing agenda is to be successfully developed at the team level, it can only be achieved through a process of open and equal communication with all team members, of all professions. Teamworking skills are clearly important for this, and the emphasis on these skills in nursing training must be an asset here. However, open and equal communication cannot be guaranteed by team skills as they are normally understood. Another dimension needs to be added to teamwork. Certain principles need to be established and built into team norms, to ensure that the required kind of communication is achieved.

One such set of principles is to be found in Habermas's (1991) 'Communicative Ethics'. Habermas developed this system of communicative principles as a way of importing Kantian rationalism into discourse and decision-making. He sees dishonest, inauthentic and oppressive communication as characteristic of late modern capitalism, and argues a need for a communicative ethic to counterbalance this, based on Kantian rationalism but taking account also of our knowledge of psychology and interpersonal processes. Habermas's requirement, that discourse should be comprehensible, true, normatively appropriate and sincere, seems naively simplistic at first sight, but in fact it excludes a huge amount of communication characteristic of contemporary western society. All strategic and tactical communication, all stratagems in argument and manipulation of relationships are ruled out. Communication approaches that deliberately use knowledge of psychology to achieve non-rational persuasion are likewise unacceptable. The essence of Habermas's approach is that it maintains the open and rational nature of decision-making, while at the same time ensuring respect of the subjective experience of each individual involved. On a more detailed level Jannsens and Brett (1997) have developed a template for team communication that reflects and operationalises many of Habermas's principles. This includes equality of respect and importance, openness in acknowledging differences, and explicit decision rules. Although intended for transnational teams, these are highly relevant to teams in the present context.

The team and the organisation

I have suggested that a team may well develop its own purposes and its own agenda in terms of service delivery. When these team agendas are simply elaborations of the overall purpose of the organisation, there is no reason to expect problems. However, a team agenda can grow beyond the confines of the organisation's goals and constitute a potential or actual challenge to the organisation.

This is a characteristic of the 'front line' situation identified by Smith (1979) where the team in direct contact with service users develops a culture and agenda that is at variance with the 'headquarters' culture of the organisation as a whole. Sometimes this agenda falls short of the organisation's goals and the team can be seen as a block to the organisation delivering its services to users. Sometimes however the team agenda goes beyond the organisation's own agenda and seeks to draw on the organisation's resources and legitimacy to develop an extended or elaborated service. The organisation has a right to require its front line teams to carry out its agenda in terms of service delivery at a standard required by the organisation. It exists to do this and it can apply that principle to all its component parts. But West (1997) argues that teams are able to be creative in carrying out the purpose of the organisation, and improvements in service delivery are often initiated by innovative teams. For such a team to challenge the practices of the organisation may in many cases be a means whereby practices are changed to improve service delivery. The trend toward loose permeable organisations of the kind described by Meads and Ashcroft (2000) probably makes it easier for teams to strike out on their own, because internal norms and procedures of control and surveillance will be weaker; but it will also make it more difficult to predict what influence this will have on the rest of the organisation, than in more traditional bureaucracies. In this context a degree of sure-footedness in organisational terms will be a considerable asset for members of innovative teams.

Teamworking across organisations

Inevitably the inter-organisational team will have a rather different identity from a team that is located entirely inside an organisation. As Ovretveit (1993) points out inter-organisational teams also need to make use of a wider variety of structures, particularly in terms of the accountability of the individuals within it. It will be more difficult to establish a set of agreed rules of operation for such a team because of the lack of a single context for negotiating and legitimising such rules. This will place greater demands on the members of such teams in terms of their ability to resolve disputes and conflicts from their own resources.

A single-organisation team only needs to concern itself with the agenda of one organisation, and that can become routinised and assumed to a significant degree. By contrast, even if the organisations supporting an inter-organisational team appear to be largely in agreement about its purpose and about the nature and extent of their commitment, the reality is that there will be a good deal of variation and uncertainty, and that the mandates of individual team members will include a degree of ambiguity which cannot be absorbed within one organisation. This is a familiar experience in the contemporary NHS where as Sheaff (1999) describes, recent policy developments leave large areas of vagueness that require those implementing that policy to fill in the gaps of their own resources. The task of team members in clarifying their role as a team is therefore a good deal more complex, and, what is perhaps more important, the responsibility to do this is a good deal more onerous. In a sense we could argue that team members are fulfilling their responsibility to their employer by clarifying the team's role, and their role in it. But the reality is that the combined or interlocking purposes of the organisations involved may not constitute a coherent agenda, and that the team must to some degree recast that agenda to become coherent. This again will make considerable demands on the team's ability to operate in accordance with good team practice and communicative ethics.

The issue of political legitimacy constitutes a major fault-line under the interorganisational team, and could become a source of tension within the team. I suggested above that organisations in the NHS have a very different legitimacy base from local authorities, and in some ways the base is weaker, in that local health bodies must look to central government for legitimacy, whereas local authorities have a direct relationship with their local electorate. Where conflict arises in the team, legitimacy may well be an issue, explicitly or implicitly, and those team members who can claim to be working to a local authority agenda will generally have the strongest claim to local political legitimacy for that agenda. This could present a difficulty for nurses, as employees of local health bodies. It could be argued that central government, which has ordained most recent interorganisational activity in health and social care, is the only true source of legitimacy for this in any case, as it is the purposes of central government that are being expressed, and both trusts and local authorities are its instrument in this. This provides health workers with a general source of legitimacy. However, I argued in Chapter 3 that nurses need to develop their own health care agenda that does not simply reflect that of the government, though it needs to connect with it.

Conclusion

In the end the problem of political legitimacy is insoluble for as long as health care is run by bodies with only token local representation. This problem is likely to be a continuing source of friction between and within organisations, and within teams, and nurses are likely to experience this in an uncomfortable way. For the nursing profession to cast itself purely as an instrument of central government policy would not be helpful. The main alternative source of legitimacy, a workable consensus on the nature and priority of health, is a more appropriate goal for nursing.

6

Nursing and other professions

Introduction

This chapter discusses the significance of professions in health care, and compares nursing with two other key professions – those of medicine and social work. The comparisons focus on the values and ethics of the three professions, and their mechanisms of regulation. The implications of interprofessional practice and of convergence between professions are considered.

Professions and codes

The importance of interprofessional teamwork in the NHS is paramount, and if we are to manage this process successfully, we need to understand something of the professional differences that provide the background to that process. Professions constitute a major component of the power structure of the health care system in the UK, as in most advanced societies. They provide a counterbalance to the power of state bureaucracies, and, in the case of one profession, medicine, have exerted a countervailing power of great significance. The function of professions as social institutions has had a good deal of attention from sociologists during recent decades, producing a range of models (e.g. Freidson 1970; Johnson 1996). These have in common a view that professions are important instruments for establishing and perpetuating the power and status of particular occupational groups. Because of the autonomous elements in their structure and functioning, professions have been able to resist to varying degrees the desire of state and other bodies to control the activities of their members. Some professions are better at this than others, and those that are most successful are usually those with the most extensive control over entry, standards of training and practice. Those professions with formal regulatory bodies overseeing practice with the power to expel practitioners from the profession are the most successful in terms of independence. In health care the medical profession has been particularly successful at establishing both power and independence. Nursing has had a more modest measure of success in this respect. Both of these professions can be contrasted with an occupational group such as social work, which had no regulatory body until 2001. In the cases of both nursing and medicine the regulatory bodies have produced codes of conduct that provide an ethical basis for professional standards.

The status of the code of professional conduct is inevitably linked with the status of the body promulgating that code, and both the NMC (as successor to the UKCC) and the General Medical Council (GMC) represent a particular kind of relationship between their profession and the state. The bodies are set up by statute, have statutory powers in relation to their professions, and perform their function on behalf of the state. But they are independent of government. I suggested in Chapter 3 that this arrangement could be seen as a contract between the state and the profession. On the other side of the equation we could also see, in the case of nursing, a contract between the individual nurse and the NMC. The nurse registers, and by doing so commits herself to the standards of the professional body, and specifically to its code of conduct. In return the NMC ensures that all other nurses are practising to that level; something that is in the interests of each individual nurse to maintain. So the code of conduct represents the contract both between nurse and professional body, and between professional body and state, the latter two acting on behalf of the patient. I have argued elsewhere that the nurse's obligation to observe the code is based on an implicit promise, represented by the fact of registering (Wilmot 1998). In one sense it is a promise to the professional body, but that body is acting on the patient's behalf, so in another sense it is a promise to the patient. Clearly most patients will not know the contents of the code, and may well not know of its existence, but the code is in the public domain, and in that sense the nurse's promise is a public promise. That provides a basis for an obligation to observe the code. The same reasoning could be applied to the GMC and its code. In each case the body issuing the code also has regulatory power over professional conduct, and in the case of nursing the code of conduct provides an explicit basis for its review of cases of unprofessional conduct. So the code is also enforceable. But its enforceability only provides a prudential reason for observing the code (to avoid being struck off the register). My argument above is that the idea of the contract provides an ethical reason for observing it.

The function of the codes of these professions can be contrasted with the situation in social work, where the historical absence of a regulatory body has led to a rather different situation. One effect of this has been that other bodies have sought to define the necessary standards of social work, in accordance with their particular interests. Employers have sought to do this, in different ways at different times in the history of social work. Those involved in training social workers in higher education have likewise sought to do this, often with a very different agenda from that of employers. A professional association, the British Association of Social Workers, has attempted to do this by producing a code of ethics for social workers (BASW 2002). But in some ways the nearest equivalent to the NMC in social work has traditionally been the Central Council for Education and Training in Social Work (CCETSW), a state-financed body responsible for the training of social workers. Because of its specific remit it was not equivalent to the nursing body, as its only regulatory power was over training, not over individual practitioners. But it is significant that Hugman and Smith (1995) use CCETSW's paper 30 (CCETSW 1991) as a definitive source on Social Work values, very much as a nursing or medical writer would use the professional code. This situation has produced a very different overall picture in relation to social work, as compared to nursing and medicine. In particular, as there has been until very recently no identified body standing as the link between the state and the profession, it has been more difficult for the social work profession to establish a coherent identity.

However, this situation is changing, as the new General Social Care Council began its work in 2001 (Department of Health 2001). Like the NMC, this body is part of the labour government's agenda of modernising professional regulation, but unlike the NMC it is taking over a previously unregulated profession. In due course, if this body operates effectively, we might expect a degree of convergence in formal machinery between nursing and medicine on the one hand, and social work on the other hand. Whether this leads to other kinds of convergence is harder to predict, although it is clear that other processes, such as the beginnings of shared training, are also working in this direction.

Medicine

I said earlier that medicine has provided a significant countervailing force to the state in the development of health care during the twentieth century and its power has significantly shaped government actions and decisions relating to health care. According to Klein (1995), the power of the medical profession constituted a major constraint for Bevan in his creation of the NHS in 1948, and it has exerted considerable power, both persuasive and coercive, in the years since. In the context of this discussion it is misleading to speak of professions as if they were largely equal to one another. The political truth is that the professions in health care include medicine, which retains a disproportionate degree of power and status; and the rest, which do not; and that nursing, despite its preponderance in terms of numbers, is one of the rest. So it is important from the point of view of nursing to have a clear view of the origins of medical dominance. To some degree these can be seen as a political process whereby a particular alliance of groups which came to make up the medical profession developed a number of power bases during the period from the mid nineteenth to the mid twentieth century. As Blane (1997) describes, the position of autonomy and monopoly attained during this period was achieved partly through political lobbying, partly through threats of industrial action and boycott. The supposed superiority of medical knowledge in terms of its scientific basis has enhanced the status of medicine during the twentieth century, but it does not adequately explain its rise to power in the nineteenth century, when the scientific base of medical knowledge was very limited and much medical treatment was ineffective. The political skills of the leaders of the medical profession were probably a good deal more important than the medical skills of doctors in explaining their rise to dominance. This showed itself in the development of medical autonomy and monopoly, but also in the success of the medical profession in influencing and to some degree controlling the development of the other professions such as radiographers (Larkin 1983).

By the time the NHS was created, the medical profession were in a position to negotiate on virtually equal terms with Bevan, the Minister of Health, on their role in the new service. It is an indication not only of the political power of medicine, but also of its cultural power, that the new service was created on the assumption that the heart of health care is medical care, and that the appropriate model of the National Health Service should be a hospital-dominated system for delivering medical care to the sick. Part of the equipment of the medical profession in its shaping of health care is the biomedical model of health, discussed in Chapter 1, reflecting the medical profession's view of health. The dominance of this model of health, together with the power of the medical profession, meant that the culture of the NHS for at least its first two decades reflected a reactive, illness-centred approach to health care (Ham 1999). Hospitals and hospital consultants controlled the bulk of the resources of the NHS, as they had dominated medicine since the nineteenth century. This structure was not suited to overall planning, rational prioritising or the proactive promotion of good health. It tended to be uncoordinated and expensive, and this did not change very much until the 1970s when the growing resource hunger of the NHS led governments to reconsider its structure and start to encourage planning, prioritising and an element of management rather than mere administration. This can be seen retrospectively as the beginning of the challenge to medical dominance, though at that stage it was implicit rather than explicit. More determined attempts to introduce management values into the NHS in the 1980s continued the process, as did the reforms of the 1990s. This was accompanied by cultural changes in public and professional perceptions of health, and a retreat of the biomedical model in favour of a more holistic view of health.

The present situation presents a picture of a profession that retains a strongly entrenched position, and remains the most powerful force in health care after the state. However, it has lost some ground culturally, in terms of the perception of the community as a whole. In the machinery of health care there is a clear challenge by other groups, particularly by managers, but by the other professions also. This should not be exaggerated, however, as Dent (1995) points out. There are numerous situations in health care where the doctor is still clearly the most powerful figure in the picture, and managers, nurses, and other participants struggle to balance this.

Medical ethics and values

We have considered how three professions are organised, and how their codes of ethics or codes of conduct represent the role of particular professional bodies in relation to the state and the patient. We have not yet considered how those codes might reflect the ethical tradition and culture of the professions concerned, and how we might understand these in an interprofessional context. We need to do this now. We also need to consider what other aspects of these professions might guide us in understanding their ethics and culture, and to understand the processes shaping the responses of the individual practitioner.

Nursing was considered in Chapter 2, so there is no need for a lengthy treatment here. I suggested there that the nursing code balances utilitarian and deontological ethics with something of a bias toward the deontological, particularly emphasising the uniqueness of the individual. I suggested that nursing ethics literature also places emphasis on the concept of care, as a moral principle and as a professional value. I suggested that our evidence on the values of individual nurses suggests an orientation toward duty, care and valuing the individual. And I suggested that the knowledge base of nursing is also individualistic. If we compare this profile with those of other professions with which nurses most co-operate, we may discover some significant patterns of difference.

The Hippocratic oath tells us a good deal about the ethics of medicine, not so much through its content as through the fact that it is still widely perceived as providing the ethical basis of medicine. It has functioned until very recently as an ethical affirmation for doctors. Henry (1995: p. 254) comments that though the oath as such is no longer taken, the medical profession is nonetheless bound by a duty to the 'principles and values implied within its dictum'. A modern successor, the 1946 Geneva declaration

(World Medical Association 1989) is consciously worded in a way that is resonant of the Hippocratic oath. All this is interesting, given the origins of the oath as part of a particular school of healing in classical Greece. The precise identity of that school is subject to some debate, but Edelstein (1989) makes a convincing case for identifying it with the healing methods of the Pythagorean cult. When the whole text of the oath is considered it is clear that much of it is dramatically and quaintly irrelevant to modern medicine, and indeed Edelstein argues that the Pythagoreans were something of a minority, even a marginal element in ancient Greek healing. But aspects of the oath have been taken up at different times in history, in part because some of its prohibitions accord (for non-Pythagorean reasons) with the prohibitions of catholic Christianity. These connections are entirely accidental, and if Edelstein is right, there is no moral, philosophical or cultural continuity in the meaning of the oath. Pellegrino (1989) points out its manifold shortcomings as a basis for modern medical ethics. All this suggests that medicine is somewhat ahistorical in its understanding of its own values; that it overemphasises the common features between the role of the modern doctor and the mediaeval and ancient equivalent, and underemphasizes the profound changes since the renaissance which have created medicine as a modern enterprise. To entertain the idea that medical values are fundamentally unchanged over more than two millennia, as well as being simply inaccurate, is entirely unhelpful in enabling doctors to develop their practice and their ethics in the context of a late modern social environment.

The Declaration of Geneva (World Medical Association 1989) as an attempt to rewrite the Hippocratic oath for the modern world retains aspects of the original that can be seen as reflecting something of the reality of medicine, and perhaps helping to mould that reality. The most salient characteristic is an emphasis on the doctor as a member of a special category, a body of brethren for whom the moral demands of medicine require a special degree of self-discipline. The message of the code is that it is incumbent on individual doctors to live up to the rigorous requirement of the profession, and apparently to do this in relative isolation. This isolation is to some degree perpetuated in the language of the most recent code available to doctors in the UK, the GMC duties of the doctor (General Medical Council 2002). Here again there is only a very limited acknowledgement of shared practice and shared decisions.

This can be contrasted with the nursing code, where the responsibility of the individual nurse is also emphasised, but the nurse's duty to co-operate with colleagues, other professionals, organisations and others involved with the patient is given considerable weight. The importance of equal, co-operative relationships in nursing comes through very strongly in the nursing code, and the contrast with the GMC code is evident. In nursing professional obligations are seen as a uniting factor, bringing people together, whereas in medicine they seem to be seen much more as an individual burden.

However, these differences are in part a matter of language and emphasis, and in other respects there are important similarities. The areas covered by the GMC code are not greatly different from those covered by the nursing code. In that sense the issues that matter to the two professions are similar and what is required of practitioners is also, in literal terms, not greatly different. There may be some convergence here, as the difference between the nursing code and the Declaration of Geneva is very marked, whereas the more recent GMC code comes considerably closer, in tone and content, to the nursing code.

If the codes of the medical profession seem to have a narrower focus than those of nursing, the literature of medical ethics has a broader focus. This however, does not necessarily mean that doctors have a broader ethical perspective than nurses. The development of the medical ethics literature base has taken a rather different course from that of nursing, in that the territory of medical ethics shades over into a larger area known as bioethics, and this in turn is part of a larger area still, that of health care ethics. Nursing ethics literature is also part of the literature of health care ethics, but it is a more clearly discrete part of that wider field. Medical ethics is not a discrete area by comparison, and it is impossible to divide off a clear body of literature as exclusively medical ethics, as can be done with nursing ethics. Medicine has suffered by its particular status, in this area, in that it has been 'colonised' by ethics writers from outside medicine – often philosophers, theologians and lawyers – who have developed the literature of medical ethics into the bigger (but still medically focused) field of bioethics. This colonisation has not been such a pronounced feature in the UK as in the USA, where Martensen (2001) sees it as a key aspect of the recent history of bioethics. Bioethics literature shares with nursing ethics literature the use of the 'grand theories' of utilitarianism and deontology, and the four principles of benificence, non-malificence, justice and autonomy. As in nursing ethics, different writers emphasise different aspects of these ideas. As with nursing ethics, medical ethics/bioethics literature also includes consideration of issues of virtue and character. And like nursing it includes a focus on duty to the individual patient.

However, medical ethics/bioethics includes a much deeper and wider consideration of issues of justice in health care than does the nursing literature. This relates back to a point made in Chapter 2, that nurses have shown relatively little interest in issues of rationing and prioritising in health care, arguably because they have had little power over this. By contrast the medical profession has had a good deal of power over these issues, and they have featured widely in the medical ethics journals and texts. However, the fact that their ethics literature has been expanded by academics from outside medicine means that we cannot assume that what is in the literature necessarily reflects the ethical repertoire of doctors in practice. And there is some evidence that at least one sector of medicine, general practitioners, are not comfortable with rationing. Ayres (1996) found that GPs were not happy with the rationing implication of fundholding, and other writers such as Toon (1994) and Smith and Morissey (1994) have suggested that the rationing role conflicted with the tradition in medicine of duty to the individual patient. Another perspective on this issue is offered by Hope *et al.* (1993) who suggest that doctors engage in covert rationing decisions disguised as clinical decisions. Hope *et al.* suggest that there is some unclarity in the thinking of doctors on this issue, and we may suspect that that unclarity is actually a result of the discomfort felt by doctors about the idea of rationing as such. So although in one sense doctors do have more experience in this area than nurses, that has not necessarily equipped them as well as it might have done to deal with the demands of rationing and prioritising. For both professions, then, this remains a problematic area.

The other difference between medical ethics and nursing ethics is that the concept of care, which constitutes an important component of nursing values and ethics as expressed in the literature, does not feature nearly as strongly in the medical context. There is a strand of writing in medical literature that does focus on the doctor-patient relationship as the crucial part of the transaction, represented by writers such as Neighbour (1997). This can be linked to what Seedhouse (1991) calls the 'carer' strand in medical behaviour – one of four strands, the others being labelled by Seedhouse as 'mechanic', 'purist' and 'guardian'. Seedhouse's view is that the carer perspective is subordinate in medicine, and that the mechanic (focusing on the physical processes of cure) and the purist (focusing on the scientist role in medicine) remain dominant. We might suspect, however, that the 'guardian' category, concerned primarily with public health, will become more important as the role of medical specialist in public health develops a higher profile.

What we know from research about doctors' ethical perspectives tends to suggest that the differences between the traditional values of medicine and nursing still persist to some degree, though the evidence is not unambiguous. Kuhse *et al.* (1997) did not find wide differences between the way nurses and doctors thought about ethical problems, but the differences that did exist accorded with what can be inferred from the codes and literature. Robertson (1996) found that doctors were more oriented toward intervening to maximise well-being, with a commitment to successful treatment, while nurses were more oriented toward respect of patient individuality and autonomy, and toward the care and comfort of the patient. These differences seem greater than those embodied either in the codes (at least the modern codes) or in the literature, and seem to correspond to what might be seen as the traditional differences between medicine and nursing.

We might infer from the above that medicine and nursing actually have a good deal in common in terms of their focal values. They share a strong sense of duty to the individual patient, a commitment to individual professional responsibility, and a set of mainstream ethical principles. Differences of emphasis certainly exist, and to some extent the development of health care puts pressure on both professions to compromise on their particular ethical profiles. The cultural ascendancy of the doctor, and the deferential compliance of the patient, which allowed medicine to operate in a somewhat paternalistic manner, are disappearing.

Nursing in turn may well discover a need to develop an ethics of treatment, and an ethics of distributive justice, to equip nurses for an extended role, both clinically and politically. The pattern is likely, then to be one of convergence.

Social work ethics and values

The interface with the social work profession and nursing is characterised by a very different set of contrasts. The status of social work in health and social care has always been problematic, with somewhat unclear boundaries and an equally unclear public perception of the social work task. Public uncertainty about what social workers do is accompanied by a tendency to view social work as primarily concerned with the most marginalised groups in society, something that in itself tends to depress the perceived status of social work. It is also a more recent institution than either nursing or medicine. A unitary training system only came into being in the early 1970s, and many of the activities that came to constitute social work were only established on any scale in the public sector in the late 1940s as part of the creation of the welfare state. During the period since their creation, their ability to influence the development of social and health services has been very limited, compared with that of medicine and to a lesser degree nursing.

During the 1960s there were signs that the values and aspirations of social work were in tune with that of government, academe and the general direction of national culture, toward an inclusive, caring and non-punitive society with a high value on public and state responsibility for the welfare of the individual. The high water mark of this era was probably the Seebohm Report (1968), which led to the creation of local authority social services departments. However, from the mid 1970s onward economic constraints and political and social changes have carried the tide of public opinion in the opposite direction, toward individualism in relation to economics and welfare, and to a more pessimistic and punitive view of human motivation and behaviour. According to Langan (1993) this left social work somewhat stranded in cultural and political terms. During this period social work has also undergone a steady process of public questioning as a result of a series of failures, mostly in the child protection field, which led to heavily publicised public enquiries. These developments contributed to an increased sense of marginalisation by social workers, which may reflect something of reality in their relationship with the rest of the community.

The key fact about social work that distinguishes it from medicine and nursing is the moral nature of its task. I suggested in Chapter 1 that health is not a moral good in the sense that, say, justice is, but that it is a good of a different sort, comparable in terms of its importance. In this it resembles happiness, wisdom and a number of other goods. Any of these can be recruited as a yardstick for moral good (as has been done by the utilitarians) and it is clear that the ascription of any of these to a person or situation is a commendation, but not a moral commendation. Medicine and nursing are in the business of promoting health, and are able to claim the endorsement of the community for doing this, because despite the increasing privatisation and individualisation of society, health care is still seen as (at least in part) a public good. Despite uncertainty about its nature, this still holds firmly enough to secure for the time being the public position of the two professions.

However, social work is in a different business. Its aims are more closely related to explicitly moral values – solidarity, humanity, equality, inclusion – and its concern is with those aspects of life that tend to be readily judged in terms of moral right and wrong, such as child care and family life, the care and control of the vulnerable and the deviant. There is no non-moral good equivalent to health that social work can proclaim as its goal. Also, there is nothing in social work values that is relatable to universal individual self-interest, as is health. For most people the message of social work concerns the treatment of others (generally disadvantaged minorities) rather than the maximising of their own interests. This inevitably increases the sense that social work is engaged in a moral judgement upon the conduct of society to the less fortunate. In a society where morality is increasingly seen as a private matter, and a relative matter, the identification of social work with a public level of morality makes it more difficult for social work to find a secure basis in popular culture. The image of the 'do-gooder' is hard to shake off because it represents something real.

If we consider the values of social work as expressed in its literature, we find the above picture confirmed, and the contrast with nursing and medicine sharpened. One major contrast lies in the fact that the body of ethics literature of social work is noticeably small when compared with those of the other two professions. This would seem strange for a profession for whom moral values are central to its project. However, I would suggest two reasons for this situation. One is that because social work practice is so explicitly dependent on the articulation of values, most social work literature must address values, and the need for a separate literature concerned with values and ethics is reduced. It is significant that classic social work texts such as Biestek (1957) are at least in part statements of values. However, there is also a second reason. An important function of ethics literature in nursing and medicine is to explore the ethical concepts important to those professional practices, and debate their meaning and significance. It is very much part of the ethical project in nursing and medicine for key values and ethical concepts to be questioned and analysed. For instance, while patient autonomy is seen as important value for nursing, the arguments for paternalism are explored. In social work the depth and intensity of reflection is no less – probably it is greater. But the discussion is more partisan. For understandable reasons it is difficult to find arguments against equality or inclusion being explored in the social work literature. There is no acceptable space for the role of devil's advocate to be undertaken in social work, so very little literature has developed which actually pursues this kind of questioning.

To explain this we can draw on the content of the BASW *Code of Ethics* (BASW 2002). This includes elements that are authentically different, in content as well as in language and emphasis, from those of the other two professions. For example section 3.2. expresses a commitment to social justice. Clause 3.2.2 indicates that conflicts of interest between clients and the bodies making and implementing social policy (including the state) are envisaged as part of the context of social work, and that social workers must be prepared to respond to these conflicts by challenging state and public policies where appropriate. So social work ethics, like social work values, are based on an expectation of collective conflicts of interest, and on a critique of the social and political order. Politics and ethics are not divided. This message comes through clearly from a large part of the social work ethics literature – for instance from Jordan (1990), and from Hugman and Smith (1995). This divides it from nursing and medicine, whose ethical systems contain few explicit political considerations, and whose political agendas are expressed in quite different terms.

The ethical codes of nursing and medicine operate on an assumption that agreement is possible, and that adherence to the agreed code of ethics is in the interests of everyone. In that context, it is possible to engage in intellectual analysis of ethical concepts, on the assumption that the fruits of such exploration, if rigorously conducted, can be agreed by all, in a context of shared rules of analysis. Such an activity is therefore worthwhile. However, where the context is one of conflict, and the profession is partisan in that conflict, there can be no shared process of refining and developing ethical concepts, because the intellectual framework for that activity, a shared commitment to clarity, is absent. Claims that such a shared commitment exists are seen as part of a process of denial of the reality of conflict, a kind of false consciousness. The ethics of social work are founded on an expectation of conflict, and that, I would argue, means that there is likely to be something of a problem in finding common ground with the other two professions on ethical issues.

However, as with nursing and medicine, there are signs of convergence. The consultative draft code of practice produced by the General Social Care Council (GSCC 2002) does not reflect the BASW concern with conflict and injustice. It is much more similar in tone and content to the nursing and medical equivalents. This may represent a shift in social work values, but it may equally represent the fact that the GSCC is concerned with a wider range of workers than BASW, including a greater preponderance of residential, day care and domiciliary workers. So we may be seeing the beginning of a dilution of the distinctiveness of social work within a larger workforce.

A framework for interprofessional collaboration

Interprofessional collaboration is a fundamental requirement in health care. Different areas of expertise must be brought together in order to ensure that patients receive the appropriate range of services. We can consider the process in a purely additive way, as the bolting together of different expertises and resources to meet a particular set of needs, or we can see it as multiplicative, as something which will enhance the practice of everyone involved, through the enhanced understanding they derive from interaction with other professionals. We can also see it as a process whereby the professionals can shift and overlap their boundaries, re-allocating or sharing tasks. The logical conclusion of such a process might be a radical redrawing of professional boundaries and tasks, or a merging of professions (Beattie 1995). The latter outcome would run up against the institutional power and interests of the professions involved, but a process of evolution in this direction is not thereby ruled out.

The fundamental issue in this area is the appropriate balance between diversity and homogeneity. One rationale for professionalism is that diversity allows specialisation and a high level of expertise. The advantage of homogeneity is that it allows coherence and consistency. A tried and trusted method for seeking to reconcile these two is the multiprofessional team. Depending on the functioning and organisation of the team, this structure allows for co-ordination of the contribution of members, and can also facilitate the cross-fertilisation of knowledge and skill (Pritchard 1995). All of these processes depend on the quality of communication within the team, and the way this is managed. At a technical level, effective communication and effective management are keys to these processes. However, there are issues other than the allocation of tasks and skills. The difference between professions is not simply a matter of what they do, or even of the kind of knowledge they use to inform what they do. Different professions have different cultures, different discourses, different values and different priorities.

A further question arises, then as to what the best balance is between diversity and homogeneity in these areas. It could be argued that differences cannot be justified with regard to values or culture, as it can with regard to skills and knowledge. A distinct skill and knowledge base can be seen as an asset – an extra resource to add to the team repertoire in responding to client need, and therefore increasing the likelihood that client need will be met. It is the classical economic argument for the division of labour. But can we apply the same argument to culture and values? After all, we might see different cultures and values as exclusive rather than as additive. We cannot believe two opposite things at once – at least if we do, it is not likely to be helpful to our practice. So what use are alternatives in the first place?

My argument would be that, although professional cultures and values are not additive as are skills, their potentially conflicting nature does not mean that they cannot be juxtaposed in a helpful way. I would suggest two ways in which this might happen. One is that it is always helpful to have the opportunity to review our own professional culture, values and priorities in the light of comparison with alternatives. This may enable us to clarify and sharpen our arguments in support of our own priorities, and to understand these better in the context of a wider range of ideas. It may in fact lead us to review our priorities, and to allow ourselves to be influenced by other groups. But the benefits of cross-fertilisation do not depend on convergence, and, as I shall suggest below, convergence is not necessarily the best outcome for the patient. This relates to the second way in which the juxtaposition of different professional values can be helpful. For this I shall first return to a point I have made a number of times so far – that the degree of consensus in our society on issues such as the nature of health and well-being has diminished in the past half century, and health care workers must operate with a diverse patient population in this respect. A health service workforce with a single set of values and priorities would inevitably find itself out of sympathy with some part of the patient population. But diversity of values among the professionals can match the diversity of the patient population and provide patients with points of contact and common ground. There will be those who feel more comfortable with an individualistic, paternalistic doctor, those who prefer a humanistic, person-centred nurse and those who resonate with a radical collectivist social worker. These of course are stereotypes. But they connect with authentic world-views, all of which need to coexist in the community as well as the professions.

There has been a sustained process of argument in parts of the health care system that we should be seeking to reduce professional differences and achieve a degree of convergence in health care. Indeed arguments have been put for a radical redrawing, or abolition of professional differences and the creation of entirely new structures (Beattie 1995). The argument I am pursuing here implies a cautious view of this project. A homogenisation of culture and values in the health care system has dangers. A state health care system working to a monolithic system of values would find itself at odds with a diverse society. It would also be at odds with the model of the liberal democratic state that encompasses it. Moral absolutism is a sustainable position for personal morality, but it has great dangers if it becomes embedded in state activity. However, the opposite of absolutism, moral relativism, is equally unsustainable for health care professionals. A commitment to respect all beliefs and positions in all situations may work in application to patient behaviour but it cannot be extended to colleagues. Some goals, and therefore some values, have to be shared within the team and the organisation. Some goals and values would be unacceptable in our system of health care. So we are in the position of being unable to operate the most extreme (and therefore most logical) positions on the absolute-relative continuum, and of having to find a 'middle way', which like all middle ways, carries the risk of incoherence.

In fact such a position exists, and does have an acceptable degree of coherence in my view. This is often termed 'ethical pluralism' (Larmore 1994), and works from the principle that ethical positions are not self-contained systems that are therefore impossible to compare. It is possible for adherents of different positions to meaningfully debate the strengths and weaknesses of those positions, to compare, to find shared ground and delineate areas of disagreement. It is possible also for ethical positions to be modified, and arguments to be sharpened or redirected in the light of comparison with other systems. It is essentially a dynamic approach, where absolutism and relativism are static. A pluralist approach enables the full benefits of diversity as I discussed it above, to be enjoyed, in terms of dialogue and development. I am therefore arguing that diversity is both sustainable and desirable. This diversity does not have to be dependent on a specific mix of professions. It can be based on other differences. Different organisations, different models of practice, different training courses and institutions can all carry different values and these can all contribute to a coherent pluralism in the health care system. We area not dependent on separate professions to provide this. Indeed, the disparity of power between professions has arguably limited the benefits of diversity, and it may be that there are better ways of sustaining diversity. My argument is simply that it ought to be sustained.

However, diversity must be managed, and for as long as the present disparity between the power of different professions exists, it is imperative that the worst effects of that disparity are contained and that diversity involves, as far as possible, an equal dialogue. Ethical pluralism requires, among other things, a common commitment to 'rules of engagement' between different positions, and the interprofessional team provides a concrete example of the importance of this. I set out in the last chapter the possibilities of Habermas's communicative ethics (Habermas 1991) in providing a framework for an ethical approach to team communication. The relevance of Habermas's principles can be clearly seen in the need to manage the negotiation between differing professional perspectives and ideologies.

Conclusion

The differences between the professions discussed above have deeper roots than is sometimes acknowledged, and there is no reason to suppose that the same should not be true for other professions not discussed here. However, with the necessary political will, and with the right social and cultural conditions, a great deal of change can be achieved in a relatively short time even with the most apparently entrenched institutions, such as the medical profession. Bodies that look impervious at present may prove surprisingly vulnerable in the near future. If the health and social care professions are propelled toward convergence in coming years, a good case can be made for striving to ensure that some of the existing diversity is preserved. In the case of nursing, it is particularly important that its open and flexible approach to health care is not lost in a process of homogenisation. The importance of that particular quality in nursing will become more apparent in Chapter 7.

7 Articulated consensus

Introduction

So far the following points have been made:

(1) Health is a good, the valuation of which is not in itself culture-specific. However, definitions of health are culturally variable, though with considerable overlap.
(2) The provision of health care is a value-laden activity, and those who are involved in this professionally (e.g. nurses) and politically (e.g. state and government) need to engage with fundamental moral and political issues.
(3) Cultural changes make definitions of health more problematic and the legitimacy of its provision, and providers, less secure.
(4) The nursing profession is well placed to respond to these changes, if it is able to remedy particular problems within its own culture.

This chapter places the above points in the context of the contemporary social and cultural developments often termed 'late modernity', and discusses a possible model for the development of health care appropriate to this environment. It also further develops a view of the role of nursing in this process.

Late modernity

The historical context of the health care system and the nursing profession is late modernity. The term modernity, as applied to social analysis, was first used in its contemporary sense by early sociologists such as Weber (1923) and Tonnies (1955), and is generally used to refer to the society and culture that developed in Europe between the renaissance and the eighteenth century en-lightenment, characterised by belief in the individual, in human rationality, in science, and in the development of rational and effi-cient forms of political, social and economic organisation. During the seventeenth and eighteenth centuries modernity impacted mainly on religion, science and politics, but in the nineteenth and twentieth centuries it flowered in the development of industrial economies and in the improvement of living conditions and health of the populations in modernised societies. Many of these changes were mainly the work of the large organisations, both private and public, which developed in the nineteenth century, operating on rational organisational principles and ordering the lives of large populations as employers, as government agencies and as produ-cers. During the late nineteenth and early twentieth century states and commercial organisations became increasingly skilled at assess-ing and meeting the needs, and shaping the lives of large masses of population through rationally organised mass-production, and through bureaucratic control of substantial resources. This phase of modernity is often given the label 'fordism' after Henry Ford and his particular contribution to the mass economy and the mass consumer, the Model T Ford. It was during this era that the Na-tional Health Service was created, somewhat in the fordist image. The machinery of the NHS was originally geared to delivering health care to a largely homogenous population, whose needs were broadly similar and for whom the definition of health and ill-health was unproblematic. The NHS patient would, it was as-sumed, accept what he was given, because the population on the whole accepted the legitimacy of medical definitions of health, illness and treatment, and the legitimacy of state arrangements for the delivery of these provisions.

Something rather different has emerged in the past fifty years, and it is this new situation that writers such as Giddens (1991) refer to as 'late modernity'. Economic production is no longer so widely undertaken in large conglomerations of workers producing material goods by quantity in a standardised production line. Production is now information-oriented and involves a wide range of activities, many of which are undertaken in relative isol-ation. Whether this change is in any real sense liberating for the workers is a matter of controversy. Consumption is also much more individualised, and the range of possibilities for the consumer is much greater. As Lee (1993) points out in his discussion of consumerism, this produces problems of rational choice, in that it is harder to know what consumer goods are necessary, what are useful (and in what sense useful) and what are 'luxuries' in that they perform an expressive rather than an instrumental function. These problems of choice have been compounded by the power of advertising and by the general consumerisation of culture. Advertising and other treatments of consumer goods in the media have succeeded in making it extremely difficult for consumers to make rational decisions about their needs, and about the meeting of those needs through consumption.

These economic changes toward a more individualised pattern of production and consumption are also reflected culturally in a change in the balance between obligation to others (family and community in particular) and obligation to the self. Giddens (1991) suggests that the focus on self-fulfilment and the realisation of potential reflects a shift toward greater individuality. The traditional community, still strong in 1948, seems now largely a thing of the past, a romantic memory preserved in various cultural forms such as television and radio 'soaps'. Community links and involvements are considerably weakened, partly by the individualisation of culture, partly, in Pahl's (1995) view, by the demands of work. There is evidence that the power of family ties is also weakening. The aftermath of divorce compromises family involvement for many people, and there is clear evidence, offered for instance by Davies (2000), of changing attitudes to family duty, showing a diminishing sense of obligation to help or care for relatives. The view that marriage and family-making is normal and expected – almost inevitable – has retreated and in Giddens' (1992) view has for many people been replaced by a view of domestic arrangements as vehicles for the expression of individual creativity. Choices to remain single, choices to change partners, and choices to remain childless, are all part of this pattern. The initiative in these changes is coming disproportionately from women, who have traditionally taken the greater role in sustaining the family structure, and are now developing different priorities. At the other end of the scale, involvement in politics has changed dramatically over the past fifty years, with a diminution in the number of people belonging to the main political parties, and an increase in interest-group politics in which groups and organisations campaign on single issues. Again the trend is away from standardised, mass politics and toward individualised activities.

In this context, perceptions of ethical and political principles have shifted considerably. Ethical relativism – the belief that there is no single morality but rather many moralities, and that we cannot judge one morality by another – has gained ground considerably. Ironism, the view that there is no absolute yardstick by which we can measure arguments in ethics or philosophy, is in Rorty's (1994) view the key perspective in the contemporary situation. We can link this to the increasingly diverse norms by which people live, compared with their parents and grandparents fifty years ago. This change is mainly a result of the liberalisation of western society, but it is also enhanced by the immigration of people of widely differing cultures.

This situation carries some interesting consequences for the individual in society. The majority of western economies in the modern era have been mercantile and capitalist, and these economies have given cultural legitimacy to individual action and individual responsibility, as against collective action and responsibility. Individual action has been seen as particularly important in the economic sphere, where capitalism depended on initiative and enterprise. Individual responsibility was defined to a large degree by the economic consequences of those actions – whether they led the individual and his family to prosperity or penury – and by the power of social disapproval. Tawney's (1990) classic work gives a vivid account of these values. In the late modern environment by contrast individual actions have less drastic consequences in most western societies, because people are cushioned by a greater degree of prosperity and by collective social provision. Much individual decision-making is directed, not to production or survival, but to consumption, where the consequences of decisions are of a completely different order, both of magnitude and of kind. And the power of social disapproval is much reduced. In effect the range of individual autonomy has become wider, but shallower, as a greater range of options becomes available, but of a different consequence. To a considerable degree, this is a shift from instrumental decision-making, where the individual's autonomy was geared to judgements of the prospects of survival or capital accumulation, to expressive decision-making, where autonomy is geared to judgements of personal satisfaction, pleasure, self-expression and, according to Giddens (1992), self-creation. The moral rightness of such decisions are much less likely to be a subject of judgement by others, or by the individual themselves, in this context.

Late modern health

Health as a good is defined by different people in different ways, and given that there has been variation for as long as this has been studied, it is likely that this variation will increase as our society becomes more diverse. The shape of that diversity to some degree reflects the diversification of culture generally. For one thing, health can be seen as a consumer good, and as Bunton and Burrows (1995) suggest, we can see it being consumerised alongside other goods. Healthy lifestyles, whether oriented toward diet, physical exercise or psychological and spiritual disciplines, are now available as consumer products. The authority of the medical profession no longer limits the range of treatments available, and a wide range of complementary and alternative therapies is now accessible, again as consumer products. Much of this activity can be seen as expressive rather than instrumental, in the sense discussed above. Health-related decisions made by contemporary citizens are much less likely to carry life-or-death consequences, at least in the short term, than decisions made by the inhabitants of crowded cholera-ridden cities of the nineteenth century, although the latter had considerably less information upon which to make rational decisions for survival. Many health-related decisions are expressive, in that they are geared to helping the individual define or project themselves into the world. Decisions about diet, fitness, body shape, environmental choices, are all variously connected with issues of identity and expression. And modern western cultures generate a wide range of narratives, images and models to address these areas, particularly through the mass media. As with complementary therapies, the retreating authority of the medical profession has left the field open for a multiplicity of accounts of health and healthy living.

In one area however, diversity and individuality of response is less in evidence. I refer to the increased intensity in public perceptions of health risk in certain areas. There is evidence of a changing perception of risk in western culture, and a diminishing willingness to accept environmental health risk as an inevitable part of living. Beck (1992) suggests that this is a response to the kind of health risks that modern economies produce, which tend to be 'invisible' unlike the miasmas and smogs of early industrialisation. vCJD is a good example of such a hazard, being the 'invisible' result of modern intensive food production. The possibility of developing dangerous and distressing illness such as vCJD creates considerable public anxiety where the actual risk in statistical terms seems on existing information to be very small. And yet, as Heyman (1998) points out, individual decisions to engage in risky behaviour are as much a feature of our society as public panics about health hazards. People respond quite differently to the identifiable risk of lung cancer from smoking (in that a large minority continue to smoke in presumed awareness of the risk) from the way they respond to a much smaller, less clear threat. It may in fact be the uncertainty of the risk that adds to its impact, and it seems clear that a lack of perceived control over the risk factors has a strong effect here. Heyman suggests that it is also a result of people's diminished connectedness to social relationships and networks that might absorb their anxiety and moderate their response. This increased anxiety, or reduced willingness to live with uncertainty, is in some ways the mirror image of health as an expression of expressive agency discussed above, as it represents a powerful preoccupation with self-protection and safety. It is also the opposite of expressive agency in that it tends to be associated with public panics that submerge individuality under a tide of public anxiety.

Health care in late modernity

So far I have argued that we lack a consensus on the nature of health, as on many related social and moral issues, and that this is a result of a clearly identifiable set of social developments that lie at the heart of western culture. We must now consider what are the implications of this for the health care system, and for the nursing profession. I shall start with the health care system. In the UK we have what is effectively a single state system of health care, with a much smaller private sector alongside. The state system disposes of huge amounts of taxpayers' money in a way that affects the well-being of virtually every citizen. It is therefore of supreme importance in a modern state that such as system has legitimacy; that is, that it is perceived by the citizens who pay for it to have a right to be doing what it is doing. An institution with legitimacy need not be particularly popular, nor need its decisions be so. If the population believe that it is the proper body to be doing what it is doing, then it is legitimate. In a well-functioning democracy even very unpopular governments can be seen as legitimate because they are in power as a result of the proper functioning of the system, and will doubtless be removed in due course through the same processes. Where government loses legitimacy, the state loses a vital element of stability.

Weber (1978) was the first commentator to give extensive consideration to legitimacy as an issue in its own right. He identified a shift from premodern times where legitimacy was based on tradition, to the more modern situation where it is based on 'legal-rational' foundations reflecting the rational acceptance by citizens of the need for an efficient administration and equitable legal system. Clearly acceptance is only rational for as long as the system is efficient and equitable, and that can be said as much for the NHS as for the state as a whole. Habermas (1976) has recast the legitimacy issue as a question of the state's ability to provide benefits for citizens to offset the deeply disempowering effect of the modern global capitalist economy for the individual citizen. Again, the same question can be applied to the NHS. How will it retain its legitimacy as society changes and consensus retreats, given that those changes affect health as much as they affect any other social good? How can the NHS address the needs of such a wide range of health agendas within the community?

At the moment there are a number of voices expressing anxiety. Davies (1999) argues that there is an erosion of public trust in the NHS, and uses the concept of social capital to focus this argument. Social capital is largely coterminous with public trust, but also includes commitment to support an institution, in the belief that that institution will in turn provide support when required. Welsh and Pringle (2001) identify the cause of the problem as a run-down of social capital accompanying the run-down in human and physical capital in the NHS over many years. This does not in itself deprive the NHS of its legitimacy. It is possible for an institution to be mistrusted and still be seen as legitimate. However, in late modern societies without the sustaining norms of deference and community cohesion, it is unlikely that that situation will last for long. Mistrust must lead to a loss of legitimacy. This is exacerbated by structural weaknesses in the institutions of the NHS. Mays (2000) argues that there is already a legitimacy problem, arising out of the organisational structure of the NHS, which lacks legitimising links to public involvement and public sentiment. There is no doubt that the British public are still deeply attached to the NHS, as evidenced by Hutton (2000). That must act as a counterbalance to the problems I have identified. But it is a wasting asset.

Consensus on health and health care

In order to consider responses to the issues of consensus and legitimacy, I propose to step back from the immediate health questions and consider a wider context. John Rawls (1993) has acknowledged the lack of consensus on crucial issues in western societies, and has questioned how far the enlightenment model of the liberal society, underpinned by a shared commitment to liberty, can survive in a situation where some communities do not place such a premium on individual liberty. In multicultural societies such as the US and Britain, there are communities whose cultures are underpinned by priorities different from those of the majority, often priorities that are less individualistic and more collective, prioritising duty and solidarity above individual liberty. In a society where such a range of priorities exists, how are we to achieve the kind of shared commitments that are necessary for a democratic political system to work? Rawls argues that a different kind of liberalism is needed to respond to the challenge of plural societies. He calls this new version of liberalism 'political liberalism' to distinguish it from traditional liberalism. He distinguishes political values from other values and argues that it is possible to have agreement on one key political value even when there is great variation in the 'comprehensive conceptions of the good' by which people conduct their lives. That key political value he believes to be justice, and he argues that it is possible to believe in a rational definition of justice from a number of different standpoints, reflecting different general value systems. He refers to this phenomenon as overlapping consensus. He argues that he has already to some degree mapped out a rational definition of justice that is freestanding in terms of general value systems (Rawls 1971). He offers the example of that definition of justice being arrived at by way of a religious view of freedom of faith and also from a different starting point, that of Kantian rationalism. Rawls does not argue that it is possible to arrive at a shared view of justice from absolutely anywhere on the philosophical and religious map. He states as a proviso that the starting points need to be essentially rational. There are, he argues, many rational views as to what constitutes a good life, so this requirement need not be seen as excluding ordinary people's real-life commitments from Rawls' somewhat abstract argument.

Rawls developed this argument specifically for the sustaining of liberal democracy in a plural society, using the keystone of justice. Its relevance to health care is not a simple matter, and needs some exploration. Health is not a moral or political value as is justice, and does not have the logical features that in Rawls' view allow justice to be freestanding within differing value systems. Also, a shared view of justice is the essential cement that can hold plural societies together in a liberal polity, whereas health is simply one of a number of values pertaining to the good life that have to be negotiated in that plural society. Its status is very different from that of justice. In a literal sense there is probably a great deal of overlap in differing views of health, and a good deal of common ground between different groups, but that situation falls somewhat short of Rawls definition of overlapping consensus. By that definition, overlapping consensus does not involve compromise. Every community and value system can embrace the same version of justice fully and wholeheartedly, for their own specific reasons. It is the unique status of justice that allows this situation. By contrast, health looks as if it belongs as part of those 'comprehensive conceptions of the good', which outside of justice, do not, and cannot overlap. In that case, how are we to develop a health care system that has secure legitimacy in a plural society? That legitimacy requires a degree of consensus, which seems beyond our reach.

This challenge has been taken up by Ezekiel Emanuel (1991) who offers a political and moral framework, in the US context, for operating health care in a society with diverse health beliefs and priorities, in such a way that the system as a whole has legitimacy in the eyes of the population as a whole. He adopts a model he calls liberal communitarianism, which encompasses a multiplicity of health care schemes serving different communities. These communities are often geographical neighbourhoods, but can also be non-geographical communities of interest and belief – communities of people who see themselves as having a shared vision of health and shared priorities and needs. Many such schemes will be set up to serve ethnic communities, communities of common religion and communities of common interest in other ways (e.g., gay and lesbian communities). The system will operate on an opt-in basis so individuals will be able to choose which community, and therefore which scheme, they sign up for. Each scheme will reflect the priorities of that community in terms of its provision. Emanuel is particularly concerned with the way in which schemes are set up and conduct their business, as he sees this as the crucial reflection of overlapping consensus. There is no need for overlapping consensus on the nature or priority of health, or on specific health priorities. We take it that this cannot be achieved. Overlapping consensus resides in the process that is consistent and transparent across the whole health care system, and it is this process, rather than the outcomes in each case, that gives the system its legitimacy in the eyes of the population. From their widely different value bases, the diverse communities within that system must agree on the process as fair. This will provide the overlapping consensus.

Can we imagine such a system working in the UK? Emanuel's model seems to bear some resemblance to the version of pluralism that Parekh (1998) advocates for multi-cultural Britain, in which society becomes a community of communities, with an agreed political culture to which all communities can subscribe. But we need to consider the differences between American and British societies that may affect the 'fit' of Emanuel's model in the UK. First, America is characterised by large groupings of distinctive culture and strong identity in a way that the UK is not. As Fuchs (1990) points out the US population consists of large ethnic minorities – WASP, 'ethnic', hispanic, black, asian, jewish – and a range of religious affiliations which partly match and partly cut across the lines of ethnicity. Religion has a substantial hold on the beliefs and values of many Americans, and this shows no sign of retreating. Indeed Grantham (1998) reports it to be a growing force. Also, other kinds of group affiliation provide powerful political cement, whether this is race, gender, ethnicity or sexual orientation. Identity politics, as described by Gitlin (1993) is a powerful factor. American communities are animated by a clear ethnic, religious or other social identity, underpinned by a narrative of argument and reflection which is at least in part, rational. Also Americans are accustomed to coming together on a voluntary basis for a wide range of purposes. It is not difficult to envisage the population of the US being able to organise themselves into groupings of interest and culture, and to commit themselves to these. The other major relevant feature is that community activity and affiliation on a neighbourhood basis remains a strong feature of American society, politically as well as socially. Emanuel discusses the 'town meeting' as an accepted and credible forum for localised decision-making on major issues. This is a strong institution in parts of the United States. Finally, Americans are accustomed to the multiplicity of health schemes that their health care system generates, and to the complexities of choosing between them.

We can see some similarities between British and American societies. In the UK as in the US ethnic and other minorities have become more important in society as a whole in recent decades, are more self-confident and have a greater impact on the overall social balance. Ethnic minorities, despite their disadvantages, have had a real impact on the culture of the majority population, particularly the young (Hewitt 1986). They have also developed distinctive political agendas. This is true of other minorities who have only emerged as such in recent decades, in particular the gay and lesbian population, many of whom see themselves as a distinctive community with a distinctive culture. In addition the national minorities of Scotland and Wales have developed a more explicit political identity with the recent arrival of devolution. The population of Northern Ireland have always had that, with or without devolution.

However, minorities form a much smaller proportion of the total population than in the US. Ethnic minorities form, by contrast with the US, only 7 per cent of the total (Carvel 2001) and it is with the majority that the differences from the US lie. In some senses the white English majority of the British population has become more homogenous over recent decades, as class differences have diminished, and a middle-class lifestyle has become characteristic of many more people, alongside the development of a smaller, very disadvantaged underclass. But other processes have occurred which tend to move things in the other direction. The consumerism that has contributed to one kind of homogenisation has also created a widening of options in terms of lifestyle and daily experience. Working patterns have become much more variable. Family structures are now more diverse. This increased diversity has been accompanied by a weakening of community links and loyalties. To some degree changing working practices have contributed to this, as leisure time diminishes for the money-rich and time-poor part of the population (Pahl 1995), and leisure becomes a matter for consumer choice rather than community involvement. At the same time, organised religion, which provides a moral cement for many American communities, is retreating rapidly in the UK. Finally, there is very little experience of making the choices involved in selecting and committing to a distinctive health care programme. For most of the British, the NHS has been all there is since 1948.

For these reasons the concept of liberal communitarianism is more difficult to apply in British society, and to British health care. Much of the diversity within the British majority is a reflection of the diversity of consumer experience, rather than the diversity of communal reflection and interests. Consumer gratification is clearly shareable, but it does not in itself provide a basis for rational reflection (Lee 1993), or for ongoing community relationships. So it is difficult to envisage communities or networks of middle-class British suburbanites achieving the social cohesion or the clarity of shared belief and commitment necessary to legitimise a particular health care provision. This does not apply necessarily to the more organised minorities in the UK who could perhaps move significantly toward deciding their own health priorities, given an appropriate framework. They could probably also engage in a dialogue with one another to arrive at agreed principles reflecting overlapping consensus. In that respect they approach more closely to the American situation. But a liberal communitarian system running alongside the NHS to serve those minority groups would be constantly at risk of marginalisation, underprioritising and underfunding in an overall health care field that would remain state-dominated. The legitimacy problem would not be solved and minorities would remain disadvantaged. We need a solution for the system as a whole.

Articulated consensus

If British society and culture cannot provide the conditions for citizens to negotiate their health-related values and interests themselves, and I am suggesting that for most citizens, they cannot, then the alternative would be for the health care system to perform this function itself. Part of the response must be structural. In institutional terms there are strong arguments, particularly by Hutton (2000), for a structure that is far more democratic than the existing NHS and I considered this briefly in Chapter 5. However, it is unlikely that this will be enough on its own. Democratic bodies need to be formally and visibly representative. But to achieve legitimacy they also need to operate within a shared framework of beliefs about the nature and the significance of their business. Where such a framework is lacking, the danger is either of apathy and cynicism, or of 'majority rule', where numerical majorities do not command legitimacy. The drawbacks of the latter situation have been amply illustrated over most of the twentieth century in Northern Ireland. This is not to argue against greater democracy in the system, as it is clearly necessary. My argument is that that is not enough and that the shared framework to support the democratic institutions also needs working on.

What is necessary is that a dialogue is achieved in the interface between the health care system and the rest of the population that enables the development of a workable consensus about the nature of health, the values of health and the values that should imbue health care provision. The possibility of the population engaging with the health care system in developing a consensus over these issues depends on the health care side of the interface, and therefore on those parts of the system with whom the population are likely to be in contact. I am suggesting that the need is for consensus about the *process* related to health, a consensus about how we get there rather than where we arrive. This may well require some overlapping in the Rawlsian sense, but as its concern is with process rather than outcome, I shall use a different term to refer to it. For the rest of this discussion I shall refer to 'articulated consensus', that is, consensus that is interconnected and flexible. In relation to health and health care this consensus would be less concerned with the precise agreed definitions of health. It would be more concerned with the general field of experience that we can agree to bring into discussion of health and the kind of values that we can agree to regard as legitimate in considering the priority of health and health priorities, on both the individual and the collective levels. The achieving of this kind of consensus would be one major source of legitimacy for the health care system. It would not solve the problem on its own because there are legitimacy issues around the way health care is structured and organised (Mays 2000). But the structural problem must be the responsibility initially of government. Articulated consensus is a goal which is realistic for health care professionals to pursue independently.

We need therefore to look to the personnel at the interface who will sustain this dialogue. To some degree the task must be distributed among the professionals who work at that interface, and the assets and strengths of all those involved (especially medicine and nursing) need to be used. However, it is also true that the nursing profession has a major role to play because nursing has crucial assets in this situation. If we look at the values and skills characteristic of nurses and nursing, we can identify a good deal of what is needed to sustain this dialogue. These can be enumerated:

(1) Ability to assume a position of equality of esteem with the other. There is no tradition in nursing of seeking patient deference. While medicine seeks to shake off the persistent residue of its traditional status, nursing has a relatively clean slate. Its traditional lack of power and status is an asset in a situation where the dialogue must be one of equality. Given the shape of contemporary culture, deference and status differences can no longer provide an engine of consensus.

(2) A fundamental commitment to autonomy. This relates closely to point (1), but balances equality with liberty. It is clear from nursing literature that nursing is centrally committed to patient autonomy in its full, instrumental sense, supporting patients in making difficult and important decisions about their survival and quality of life. However, nurses are also sensitive to the expressive side of patient autonomy, relating to comfort, recognition and self-expression. In that sense they are able to respond to the full range of autonomy as experienced by people in contemporary society.

(3) Experience and skill in acting as interpreter between the patient and the rest of the health care system. This is clearly

an important part of the nurse's role in many situations, and inevitably tends to be applied primarily to issues of individual care and treatment.

(4) A commitment to the process as well as the content and outcome of the transaction with the patient. A focus on the relationship with the patient is deeply embedded in nursing thinking and practice, and this is seen as being important in itself and not simply as a means to an end.

(5) An ability to work with health as a problematic concept rather than as a firm 'given'.

These characteristics all provide a basis for the nursing profession to play a central role in the dialogue that I am outlining. The last of the list reflects Seedhouse's (2000) view that nurses are well suited to address the question 'what is health?'

To some degree this role would be an extension of the role which nurses play at present, that of explaining to patients and relatives the processes and meanings of the events they are experiencing in the NHS. It would also be an extension of the educational role that nurses already play in relation to health promotion and community health. Most of the interaction that I am suggesting for that role is already within the nursing repertoire in the community health care and health promotion role. But I am suggesting an extra dimension that would contain the following elements:

(a) A dialogue with patients, relatives and the community about the nature and value of health – what is healthy, what is unhealthy, how important is health in relation to other goods;

(b) A dialogue about what the NHS should be offering in response to their perceived health priorities;

(c) A dialogue about the desired relationship between the public and the professions and organisations involved in health care.

The crucial goal in this enterprise would be to develop a discourse through which people will be enabled and encouraged to discuss these issues as citizens, rather than simply as patients. This might involve discussion in the context of political institutions and processes – local and general elections, debates through the local media – and also private conversations between people. But in addition that discourse needs to be supported by values that optimise the quality of the interchange. I have argued earlier in the book in favour of Habermas's (1991) discursive ethics as a model for appropriate interchange between professionals and I think the same arguments apply to these encounters also. The commitment to clear, honest, equal, rational communication, expressed in Habermas's system provides the basis for the kind of dialogue needed. The five characteristics of the nursing profession that I enumerated above approximate to Habermas's model, and it follows that nurses have the wherewithal to model and encourage that kind of interchange. In terms of their skills and values, they are not unique in this respect, but in terms of the combination of skills, values, numbers and exposure at the interface between public and health service, they are uniquely placed. We cannot of course expect that nurses will of their own resources change the values that provide the rules of discourse in our society. But they can model a particular kind of discourse in a particular area.

Conclusion

If nursing is to mediate between the public and the health care system (and behind that, the state) then communicating with the public will not be enough. It will also have to communicate with other professionals, managers, politicians and academics, and I have already argued that this is an area where nursing is less equipped, and where more development is needed. Such a development would need to happen on a number of different levels, including the professional culture of nursing and the nature of its links with the other bodies it must influence. In the remaining chapters, I do not propose to consider all of these necessary developments but to focus on specific aspects. I propose to map out a possible framework for a nursing response to the health issue that would facilitate the development of an articulated consensus on health care.

8 Nurses and the public debate

Introduction

This chapter falls into three parts. The first part explores public discourse on health and health care. The second part considers further the idea of direct dialogue between the nursing profession and the general public on health and health care, first introduced at the end of Chapter 7. The third part considers the nature and potential of a similar debate at the political level, and the potential role of nursing in that context.

Key areas of debate

First we need to consider on which sort of specific issues the health debate needs to focus if we are to achieve articulated consensus.

(1) I have identified the nature of health as an area where there is no clear shared view. In a state-financed health care system the definition of health determines the range of needs and provisions that that system will resource. Is physical fitness primarily a health issue or a recreational issue? Is it the responsibility of the state health care system to promote this, and what sort of activities can it legitimately support to this end? Should sport finance and sponsorship be the responsibility of the NHS? And where should we place the boundary between health issues and cosmetic issues? Is appearance a health issue always or sometimes? Is fertility always a responsibility of the health care system, or only sometimes? These issues have all at different times been surrounded by a degree of confusion and

in some cases conflict, but there has been little evidence or progress toward articulated consensus on any of them, and in fact little coherent public debate in many cases.

(2) The importance of health in relation to other goods is another issue that needs to be addressed in this context. The UK spends less on health than most other advanced societies (Ham 1998), and yet there is no evidence that this level represents public preferences, or that the British are any less concerned about health than other nationalities. Nor is it clear that there is wide public acceptance of the full implications of greater resourcing for the NHS. There is some evidence that people will readily agree that more ought to be spent on health, and will express willingness to pay additional tax if it is hypothecated to health care. On the other hand it is not clear that the public fully accept the implications of moving resources to health from other areas of public spending (Dixon *et al.* 1997). Also there is no clear evidence that any of these views would translate into voting behaviour. The electoral success of New Labour could be interpreted as an indication that parties need to present themselves as committed to low taxes if they are to win elections. Voting behaviour is difficult to interpret, but political parties have been loath to increase taxes since 1979 and their judgement of the public mood on this issue perhaps deserves some weight. This has led to considerable caution about committing large amounts of additional money to the NHS, though that caution has relaxed with the NHS plan (Department of Health 2000) and the 2002 budget.

(3) The third area where articulated consensus is to be sought is that of health priorities, particularly in the context of rationing of health care resources. This topic is be considered in more depth in Chapter 9.

(4) The final area of importance where articulated consensus needs to be sought is that of the organisation of health care, and the distribution of power within the health care system. This includes processes of decision-making as well as structures of control. In many ways this issue is at the heart of the legitimacy problem of the NHS. Democratic control in the NHS has diminished rather than increased in the years since 1948. Decentralisation, which has happened in two major

stages since 1990 does not equate with democratisation, and has resulted in the strengthening of localised elites of managers and professionals. Mays (2000) has argued that the nature of the organisations that have been created to run health care over the past ten years have a problem of legitimacy, because of their lack of a democratic base. As with the previous issues identified, it is not clear what the public perception is of the appropriate structure and control of the NHS. The status of the traditionally dominant group in health care, the medical profession, has diminished somewhat as part of the general cultural change toward lower deference; but there is no indication that the public have identified an alternative group to whom they can entrust their care.

Public discourse on health and health care

In order to map out the context for the potential nursing role, we need to consider the process through which these issues are dealt with at present, as well as processes through which they could be addressed in the future. To do this we must look at the way in which health care issues are dealt with in the public domain. This must include the media, particularly the press and television, and it must also include those bodies that use the media and other means to address the public on health issues. Government is one of the largest generators of information on this issue for public consumption. However, other bodies with an interest in influencing the public also contribute. This includes organisations with a campaigning agenda in health care, and commercial organisations. We must consider then what kind of discourse these bodies generate.

It is clear that the media have a two-sided relationship with the health care system. They pursue an independent agenda that is often claimed to be confusing, distorting and disempowering for the public, though this is not easy to verify. Certainly media treatment of particular issues is often at odds with the agenda of the professionals and planners of the health care system. For instance Gwyn (1999) suggests that media treatment of the AIDS issue tends to play into public stereotypes of the most prejudiced kind, and their discussion of other threats to health is little short of hysterical in its oversimplifying and alarmist message. Oversimplification is also reported by Petersen (2001) in media treatment of genetic issues in health, but in this case the simplified message was one of optimism, raising unrealistic hopes. Henderson *et al.* (2000) give an example of the media agenda conflicting with that of health promotion in relation to breastfeeding, which the media portray as both difficult and deviant. But this is not a one-way street. It is clear that the media also provides a useful conduit for health promotion messages, and that many practitioners have developed skills in managing the media in order to transmit the desired message. However, the quality of that message and its impact on the public mind has been questioned. Lupton (1995) argues strongly that the way in which health promotion messages are presented through the media tend again to present a simplified message, playing upon social anxieties in a way that is manipulative rather than empowering.

One might argue that these observations simply reflect the media doing what they are good at. The task of the media in a capitalist environment is to engage the attention of the public and present its news in a way that will be understood, so that the public will feel they are getting value for money and keep subscribing. Arguably the kind of presentation described above is necessary to achieve these ends. Certainly it is clear that a strong emotional charge is important in engaging the interest of readers and viewers. It is generally true also that the media seek to identify themselves with the attitudes and prejudices of the public, and communicate through these, rather than change them. And it is clear that facts need to be simplified to be absorbed. This latter point has nothing to do with the intelligence of the public, but is simply a result of the limitations of the human brain as a receiver and store of information. It has long been understood in information psychology that information that is fragmented and complex and lacks a strong theme to hold it together will not be absorbed (see, for instance, Lin 1973). The media are struggling with this basic fact of psychology, in a situation where there are many competing foci for their audience's attention.

However, the degree of simplification necessary for the media to operate effectively makes it very difficult indeed for them to achieve a rational consideration of the issues. Rational discussion requires awareness of degrees of factual uncertainty and probability.

It also requires an awareness of the relative importance and prevalence of different problems. It requires a knowledge of context, so that specific issues can be understood as part of a bigger picture. The news media are able to provide very little of these elements, because they would get in the way of what the media need to do. It is therefore not surprising that the health debate conducted through the media is low on rationality.

However, alongside the psychological dynamic, the media are also engaged with a cultural dynamic which shapes public perception of health and public response to this, as reflectors, interpreters and transmitters of contemporary culture. In part this can be seen in the consumerisation of health and the framing of health choices as life-style options. Newspapers and magazines have exploited this trend to a significant extent. However, issues that arouse public anxiety and sometimes panic are also part of the media health diet. I suggested in the previous chapter that contemporary culture is characterised by a split attitude to risk, with an acceptance of individual risky behaviour but an increasing unwillingness to accept environmental risk and a tendency toward high anxiety where what is risked is clearly identifiable and significantly distressing. Public perception of risk is often argued to be selective, but the media are likewise selective in their treatment of risk issues. Again, media treatment of the AIDS issue, described by Kingham (1998: p. 124) clearly shows the effects of the imperatives of 'drama, conflict, controversy, human interest and brevity'. Again, we have an interactive dynamic, as the media seek to feature health issues that are most likely to arouse public interest and therefore attract viewers and readers, and these will be the issues most likely to arouse public anxiety.

We find a different picture in relation to the government's presentation of health issues to the public. A range of government documents are available to the public which, taken together, provide sufficient information, and sufficient context, to underpin a rational discussion of health issues. However, most of those documents are probably not read by the public, and in truth the public are not encouraged to read them. They tend to be read mainly by those professionally or politically involved in health care. By contrast, government use of the news media on health issues tends to operate in the way that the media themselves operate, with simplified, emotive and incomplete information. This is partly because health issues are the stuff of political debate and persuasion, and the goal is not always to inform the public but rather to persuade them to support the government. The issue of waiting lists is a good illustration of this. Although as Harrison (2000) points out, waiting lists are a relatively poor index of the effectiveness of the NHS, they have become a touchstone of success, and government has sought to gain public support with waiting list initiatives at the expense of pursuing real effectiveness in the NHS.

Other bodies present health issues to the public in ways that likewise show the limitations of their position. Commercial bodies offering health insurance and private treatment present a particular view of health in their advertising literature. This is geared to encouraging potential customers to buy their product, and carries the same caveat as all advertising. At the same time such customers are making more detailed and complex decisions than voters or newspaper readers, and so require, and usually know that they require, detailed information. Within its limits, therefore, this kind of information is often more accurate and more honest about uncertainties and probabilities than are the media and government versions of health, particularly when relating to insurance. However, they are generally concerned with fairly limited areas of health care, and are communicating to a minority of the population.

The other important group of organisations which communicate with the public on health care matters are charities and campaigning organisations, which are usually concerned with specific aspects of health, and which have specific agenda geared to gaining public support for a particular priority area or position. In many cases they are particularly effective providers of information on the issues that they are concerned with, but the information provided is inevitably partial and biased.

In general, it is fair to say that those who have an interest in providing user-friendly health care information to the public do so because they also have an agenda that involves persuading the public to vote for them, buy their product or support their cause. Those who have an interest in accessing accurate, balanced and contextualised information on health issues, such as planners, academics and politicians, have relatively little incentive to make it accessible and understandable to the public. While the available information, and the kind of opinions and analyses that sometimes accompany that information, remain partial and contradictory, this situation is not likely to change. Consensus, articulated or otherwise, is not going to be achieved in this climate.

The nurse-public dialogue

For reasons set out at the end of the last chapter, I am arguing that nurses are in an ideal position to draw the public into the above debate, and to introduce the critical, rational element which is lacking at present. As a specific methodology, I would suggest that health promotion, increasingly important to nursing, could extend into the promotion of a critical view of health and health care. How might this look in practice? After all it seems a dubious enterprise to exploit the dependence of people at a vulnerable time in their lives when they are in need of health care, and to draw them into issues that they may not wish to think about. However, taking a wider view, the imperative to empower patients by enabling them to make decisions about their own care provides a basis for empowering them also to consider in a wider context what they want from health care, and how they view their own health. Also, as I argued in Chapter 4, it is a legitimate part of the nurse's role to help the patient sustain their role as a rational citizen in the face of the pressures created by the experience of ill-health and the patient role. The important element here is not only to give information, (though that will always be necessary) but also to foster a desire for information, and a critical perspective on the information they receive. Again the existing nursing repertoire provides the resources for this in the model of adult education known as andragogy. This model is widely used in training nurses to be educators, with the work of authors such as Knowles (1990) placed alongside specific nursing applications such as that of Mast and van Atta (1986). This also provides a methodology for enabling nurses to promote health awareness in a wider sense. The theory of andragogy suggests that we are empowered through the process of problematisation; of having questions posed that enable us to think about our situation in a new way. One of the main exponents of andragogy, Paulo Freire (1972), argued that problematisation enables us to engage in a dialectical process of moving toward critical consciousness, which involves identifying the processes that underpin our situation, seeing them as dynamic rather than static, and identifying the possibilities of our changing that situation.

To problematise health is not a difficult undertaking. Individual experiences of what health 'feels' like vary significantly and there is an inevitable tension between the supposition that there is a correct, official definition of health on the one hand, and the personal experience of the complexity and uncertainly of health on the other. For the most part, that tension is denied and unacknowledged in the interface between health care providers, patients and the public. Health care is generally provided on the assumption that health is not problematic, either in its nature or in its relative importance. But the tension lurks under the surface and a modest shift in the discourse through which care is provided can bring that tension to the surface of the transaction. The tension is particularly strongly present in the field of health promotion and Duncan (1999) describes the strong awareness on the part of health promotion workers that they are not engaged in a straightforward transaction but one deeply affected by ethical and definitional uncertainties.

I suggested in Chapter 4 that it is a legitimate and indeed central part of the nurse's relationship with the patient-as-citizen to promote healthy living, and that this is sustainable from duty-based, contractarian and utilitarian points of view. I acknowledged at that point that the nature of health is problematic, but argued also that this does not in itself prevent us from working to promote health. Health remains a good in normative terms, even though its nature in descriptive terms is not agreed. However, we might wonder how it is possible to go a step further than this and promote health while at the same time actively promoting debate as to its nature and priority. It seems on the face of it a rather contradictory activity. However, I would argue that it is precisely the promoting of debate that ultimately promotes health because it enables everyone involved to own and value their own perception of health. That does not guarantee that everyone will value health above all other goods, and it is clear, again from the experience of health promotion workers (e.g. Crossley (2001a)) that this does not happen. But that is a necessary feature of a situation where people are making autonomous choices.

Skills that are widely acquired and practiced in nursing – skills of facilitating learning through an andragogic framework – need only be 'steered' to facilitate reflection on the nature of health. At the simplest level, a question 'what does it mean to you to be healthy/well' is both a facilitative part of a programme of treatment and care, and an opening-up of the debate for one individual. The framework for this process is provided by the principles and practice of health promotion, an important nursing activity of which the knowledge-base provides a workable framework for the problematisation of health. If we take the approach of Ewles and Simnett (1995), who are, in Seedhouse's (1997) view, on the more relativist wing of health promotion, it is clear that the methods they recommend would allow, indeed do allow, conceptions of health to be explored in a non-directive manner. In relation to the priority of health for individuals, Crossley (2001b) offers an interesting model for a health promotion strategy that engages with people's identity issues and moral priorities at a critical level. Those aspects of health promotion that involve working for changes in collective circumstances or lifestyle factors already implicitly raise the question of the nature and priority of health, and practitioners are likely to find themselves engaged with that question with the recipients of their service. And questions about the relative importance of health as against other goods for individuals will inevitably shade over into questions about the importance of health care for the community as a whole.

One point above all needs emphasising. These activities are an extension of what nurses already do. The terms of the discussion may have reframed those activities in a way that makes them unfamiliar, but the unfamiliarity is more apparent than real.

The political dialogue

This final section of the chapter will focus on nursing's engagement with an equivalent debate within the circle of those who control or influence health care. I shall use the term 'health complex' to refer to the occupants of that circle. We might include in the health complex ministers, senior civil servants, professional advisers to the ministers, other advisers from academic and related areas, professional organisations and regulatory bodies, health authorities, trusts and other component bodies of the NHS machinery, private providers and insurers, and interest groups of various sorts. Nursing, as a profession with a number of spokespersons in different parts of the system, clearly already has a voice, and an important one. However, nursing as an interest group is competing in this situation with a number of powerful interests. I have discussed in earlier chapters the long-established power of the medical profession in the health care system, and its several bases. That power does not simply work on the basis of the ability of doctors as a collective body to influence the rest of the health care system. It is also characterised by the presence of members of that profession in key positions in the department of health and in other bodies. However, other bodies also present significant influences, often in opposition to the doctors. Traditionally the role of universities in the health care system was to provide yet another power-centre for the medical profession. But in recent decades new health-related disciplines have produced a generation of academics who owe no direct allegiance to the health care professions and are able to provide a countervailing set of perspectives. Health care management in its manifestation as an academic discipline has been significant in this respect, as has health economics.

My agenda here is not to suggest ways in which the balance of influence can be shifted in nursing's favour, in a formal or structural sense. I am concerned with the possibilities of nursing influencing the nature of the debate on health care within the health complex, and creating a link between the discussion at this level and the discussion at the level of the general public and patients. In order to do this we need to consider ways in which we might understand the health complex in greater depth, and on the basis of that, understand how processes within it might be steered in the direction with which we are concerned with.

Pluralism and elitism

There has been a debate over a number of decades over the operation of decision-making machinery in modern democratic states. It is broadly accepted that most decision-making excludes the mass of the population, whose role it is simply to choose between two sets of political masters at intervals. There is a question however, as to how far decision-making is open to influence and pressure, at least from those parts of the population who are organised and active. Two major schools of thought exist here. One of these, the pluralist view, suggests that decision-making is open to influence by active groups within the population and that there is a good deal of competition for influence between different interest groups. The groups and organisations involved in the shaping of health care policy offer an example of this. Dunleavy and O'Leary (1987) suggest that the pluralist view has travelled some distance since the early twentieth century, when pluralists saw the political institutions of the liberal democratic state as providing the structure for a pluralist decision-making process. Neo-pluralism, by contrast, does not regard competition for influence as taking place on an equal footing, and accepts that there are disparities between different interest groups in terms of their influence. It also takes the view that formal state structures are often irrelevant to the real process of bargaining and power-broking. The essence of the pluralist view is that the process is a competitive one where debate, and jockeying for power and influence, continue and through this process, shape policy.

Effective operation in the pluralist framework involves winning supporters and creating alliances. Those operating in that framework seek to retain the essence of their particular agenda but are willing to compromise to some degree in order to find allies and tip the balance of influence. In such a situation we cannot assume a level playing field, any more than we can expect that a free market is necessarily fair or equitable in the distribution of market power. The effective operator in the pluralist framework must have a strategy for countering the effects of those inequalities in the market place of influence. The pluralist framework also requires a degree of flexibility as to who is being persuaded. Sometimes this needs to include the general public, or a part thereof. Sometimes it involves much smaller groups – cabinet, senior civil servants, key parliamentarians. In health care influential bodies needing to be persuaded are to be found in a number of organisations at local as well as national and international levels.

However, an alternative view exists as to the reality of decision-making in ostensibly democratic states. This is the elitist perspective. The elitist view is that ostensibly democratic states are dominated by small elites, generally constituting senior politicians, business leaders, and leaders of other powerful organisations, who make decisions independently of democratic processes. The elitist analysis rejects the notion of a marketplace of influence, and takes the view that the crucial discussions and conversions that determine a particular decision will take place behind closed doors, between people who have access to one another on a private and often informal footing. Socialising among the wealthy and powerful ensures that members of the elite know each other socially and are able to deal with business on a personal level. The elitist perspective sees the processes and machinery of plural debate and decision-making as being largely cosmetic, functioning to create an impression of wide consultation and persuasion, and thereby disguising the reality that power is concentrated in far fewer hands than democratic states would wish their citizens to believe.

Which is true? The problem in choosing between them is, as Dunleavy and O'Leary (1987) point out, that the two perspectives use different kinds of evidence to support their theses, and on the whole it is difficult to use evidence supporting one to falsify the other. Traditional pluralists look at the visible processes of decision-making and ask who was observed to have influenced what decision in what ways. Neo-pluralists tend to look at rather larger social and economic processes, but with a similar assumption that relevant evidence is visible to the observer. Elitists work on the basis that the real exercise of power will often be invisible to the outside observer, either because matters are settled in secret, or because that power is used not to determine the outcome between clearly stated options, but to exclude certain options from the field in the first place, so that they are never considered as possibilities in the decision-making process, what Lukes (1974) describes as the third dimension of power. The moments where the real power is exercised will be as invisible as the behaviour of sub-atomic particles, and likewise we can only observe the results of that behaviour. The elitist infers the nature of decision-making from other kinds of evidence. They look at whose interests are served by a particular decision. They also look at the connections and networks between influential individuals on several levels, family, social and institutional.

Both perspectives probably have a good deal to tell us about how things work. Given that the two maps represent rather different territories (albeit closely connected) it is not the case that we must reject one to entertain the other. However, we might ask which is more useful to provide a framework for the nursing profession to influence the health of this society.

It is clear that the two frameworks suggest very different strategies. I have already suggested the skills and priorities that might be appropriate in the pluralist framework – gaining allies, winning supporters, creating alliances and coalitions. In the elitist framework the choices are starker; enter the elite, overthrow the system, or exit the game. The health policy elite in the elitist framework would probably consist of leaders of the medical profession, senior civil servants, certain key regional and district-level figures, key academics and the leaders of the commercial sector including the pharmaceutical industry. For nursing, the goal must be to insert the leaders of the profession into the elite. They may already be there. But the historical evidence is that they have not been, and that nursing leaders have been consistently ignored (Rafferty 1992). In the very nature of elitism, it is very unlikely that outsiders will be admitted unless the elite itself wishes this. The elite may wish to accept new members either because an outsider group is dangerous enough to be a real threat to the existing power structure as a whole, or because they bring enough in the way of assets and resources to effectively buy their way into the elite. Nursing may now be sufficiently important to the government's strategy (Department of Health 1999) to qualify on the second count.

But how useful is elitism to nursing? In terms of the perspective it offers, it seems to have two opposing faces. On an individual level it chimes in strongly with the experience of powerlessness. Within this perspective decisions of any importance are beyond the reach of the practitioner to influence because we do not know that the decision is there to be made until 'the powers that be' have already decided what will happen. This scenario reflects the psychology of powerlessness that manifests itself in many occupational cultures, and is certainly detectable in the culture of nursing. A perspective that confirms and legitimises this world-view seems to be unhelpful for an empowered profession. However, at a different level elitism represents a profound political analysis wherein democratic forms are used to deceive the masses into believing that they live in a democracy, whereas real power lies with an elite representing a concentration of power. So we can be elitist for rational reasons based on political and economic analysis, or for irrational reasons based on a mixture of ego defence and maladaptive learning.

An elitist world-view based on the non-rational psychology of powerlessness looks like a recipe for doing nothing. However, the more rationally based elitist view remains a basis for revolutionary action, or for joining the elite. But I would argue that neither of these courses of action is feasible for nursing. The enterprise of nursing is based on a belief that certain interests relating to health are held in common by all citizens, and that those interests provide a basis for a degree of consensus and common commitment, whatever other conflicts of interest may run alongside these. Elitism is based on a view that the interests of the mass of the population are effectively repressed and subordinated through the operation of the elitist power structure, and that where common interests and concerns are identified, they are likely to be illusory or a matter of deception. While individual nurses may quite legitimately have an elitist analysis of power relations, it makes no sense for the nursing profession as a whole to take up this position. On the other hand the pluralist position accommodates a range of different interests that are variously reconcilable, compromisable and conflicting. It also allows for an underlying set of values that are not simply those of hegemony and domination but could also include values such as justice, equality and truth. In other words pluralist competition can operate without an assumption of irreconcilable conflict, and with an assumption of common interests. That constitutes one argument for nursing as a profession electing to operate in a pluralist framework.

We can also argue that pluralism is in accordance with the practical values of nursing in that it provides the basis for a practical strategy. Neo-pluralism does not assume consistent openness of decision-making, but it allows that such openness is possible. Elitism by contrast assumes secrecy and works on the assumption that openness is impossible. If it seems to be happening, it must be a deception or illusion. For this reason also an elitist position is unworkable for nursing. Inclusiveness and open communication are fundamental to the values and ethics of nursing, and necessary for the effective practice of nursing. It is fundamental for nursing not only that people should be involved in decisions that concern their health and their health care, but also that it is possible for them to be so involved.

Nursing and politics

We cannot assume that decision-making is open and equal in our health care system. Nurses with a pluralist approach must be prepared to encounter a good deal of inequality of influence between participants. But for a pluralist it is possible to make decision-making more open and equal than it is, through working effectively within that system. The operative word here is 'effectively'. The pluralist views decision-making as involving far more people than the elitist would allow, and this implies a much wider relevance for the exercise of political skill and judgement. The inevitable question arises, are nurses effective in their exercise of political skills? Individuals such as Florence Nightingale and Mrs Bedford Fenwick spring immediately to mind, but they are easy to identify partly because they are few and far between. The historical record must cast doubt on the political skills of nurses. The reasons for this may be discernible in the occupational culture of nursing. Degeling *et al.* (2000) offer evidence that nurses in the UK do not think politically, and are unhappy about decision-making processes involving micro-political processes of bargaining. (Interestingly, Australian nurses in this study emerged as more politically confident.) Rains and Barton-Kriese (2001) discover a similar lack of political awareness, and alienation from policy processes among nursing students in the United States.

There may be a number of things at work here, including class and gender factors. One key feature of nursing practice and culture seems particularly important however. This relates to the fact that the focus of nursing is on the private rather than the public sphere of activity. Nurses perform much of their professional activity in those parts of the patient's world that are normally regarded as private, even intimate. The nurse is permitted into that private zone, not to convert it into a public zone, but to respect its private nature. Public acceptance of this access is a great strength for nursing, but has drawbacks. Browne's (2001) comments about the influence of liberalism in nursing resonate with this emphasis on the private, non-political sphere of personal life which is strongly emphasised in liberal political theory as being an area where the state should keep out. Nursing seems more deeply affected by the private and personal world they operate in than other professions (for instance medicine and social work) who enter a similar territory, and also seems more distanced from the public, political and civic zones of activity. However, it was not always so. Nelson (2001) suggests that in the early twentieth century nursing had a strong civic focus, with a politically vocal leadership and a discourse of civic duty. So what happened? Hallam (1998), discussing the position of nurses in the mid twentieth century, suggests that following the creation of the NHS the public image and self-image of nursing shifted away from professionalism and toward a more feminised 'handmaiden' image, emphasising the personal sphere of caring. The civic tradition of early twentieth century nursing appears to have been lost in that process. Now it needs to be regained. The private and the public zones need to be reconnected by the nursing profession if it is to fulfil its potential role. A practical opportunity to start to do this is offered by the development of bodies such as primary care trusts, providing potentially useful political experience for a cadre of nurses on the boards and committees of these bodies. Whether that experience will percolate through the rest of the profession sufficiently to provide the 'critical mass' for a culture shift is impossible to predict, but it is a hopeful development.

Conclusion

An open debate is not necessarily an equal debate. Often participants differ widely in terms of resources, and those differences may well affect the direction and outcome of debate. In this context nursing always seems to be at a disadvantage where health and health care are the focus. However, a central message of this chapter is that many of the disadvantages of nursing are remediable. Potential resources to strengthen the position of nursing exist in a number of situations. These need to be realised.

9

Nurses and resource allocation

Introduction

This chapter explores the position of nursing in relation to the issue of resource allocation in health care, and compares the relative alienation of nurses from this process with the greater engagement of doctors and social workers. Several models of prioritising and rationing are considered, and the possibility of a distinctively nursing model is explored. This is discussed in the context of the main ethical principles relevant to distributive justice.

Prioritising and rationing

The issue of resource allocation, prioritising and rationing in health care has become a central concern in recent years, as the rising cost of health care and the limits on public resources have become apparent. Most considerations of the issue work from the basis that demand for health care, and the ability to benefit from it, exceeds supply and will continue to do so. Historically this is a surprise. The founders of the NHS expected that the need for health care would diminish over the years, as people's health improved and health care became more effective and more efficient. What has happened is that the traditional indices of population health, life expectancy and infant morality, have improved, but longer lives have meant a longer period spent in old age, subject to a range of health problems that place significant demand on the NHS. Medicine, and health care generally, have widened considerably the range of problems to which they can respond (although response does not always mean cure) and this has increased the cost of the NHS. The illnesses that take up much of the attention of the health care system are now chronic, requiring management over long periods. Finally, public expectations of the health service have increased a good deal over half a century. All of these things mean that the cost of health care has risen greatly since 1948. For these reasons, prioritising and rationing are major tasks for those in control of the machinery of health care at present, and for the foreseeable future.

However, for decades the issues of prioritising and rationing were hidden behind the clinical authority of the medical profession, which was assumed by the public to be making the best decisions for its patients on clinical grounds. It is only in the past 25 years, since the economic crisis of the 1970s created major difficulties for public finance, that the issue has slowly emerged into public consciousness. A crucial landmark in this process was the introduction of the internal market in 1990, requiring purchasers, particularly health authorities and fundholding GPs, to decide on the priorities that they would pursue in their purchasing policy. During the 1990s, politicians on the whole avoided the issue of rationing, sometimes to the point of denial, and responsibility for prioritising devolved to the health authorities (Court 1995). The Labour Government elected in 1997 has shown marginally more willingness to acknowledge that rationing decisions have to be made. Frank Dobson, the first Labour Health Secretary, actually made a rationing decision in relation to a particular treatment, Viagra, in 1999 (Ferriman 1999), and it could be argued that the National Institute for Clinical Excellence, set up under the 1999 Health Act, performs at least part of a rationing task. Despite the increase in the resources available to the NHS from the 2002 budget the need to ration and prioritise remains, and although we might argue that some rationing is centralised, local bodies carry a good deal of the responsibility. These include primary care trusts, which have inherited the rationing responsibilities (insofar as these have been owned) of fundholding GPs (Pickard and Sheaff 1999).

Rationing and the professionals

Nurses have had less involvement than other groups in making rationing decisions during the years when it has been part of the

agenda in NHS organisations. There are many individual exceptions to this, but those exceptions do not seem to have percolated
into the common arena of professional thinking in nursing. Nursing as a profession seems still to be relatively uncontaminated by
the rationing experience. In this respect nurses have had a different experience from at least two other professional groups with
whom they are in frequent contact – doctors and social workers.
Prioritising and rationing have had a highly ambivalent, but nonetheless important place in the recent history of the medical profession in the UK. Doctors have traditionally regarded this as the
exercise of clinical judgement rather than as rationing, but in
many cases it almost certainly shaded over into rationing decisions
(Hope *et al.* 1993). In a completely different context fundholding
GPs found themselves faced with the need to ration in order to
conserve their own fund (Smith and Morrissey 1994). The social
work experience is different again. Social workers have for many
years been in a position where they have been under pressure from
managers to conserve resources, and under pressure from clients
to provide them. Ellis *et al.* (1999) identify a widespread perception that social workers have in the past had a good deal of
discretion in making rationing decisions, relating it to Lipsky's
'street level bureaucracy' thesis (Lipsky 1980). In the view of these
writers the rationing process has been significantly more prescribed
from above since the community care reforms of 1990–93. Overall,
then, for these groups rationing decisions have been 'part of the
job' in a way that they have not been for nursing.

However, the attitudes to rationing within medicine and social
work have not necessarily corresponded with practice. In medicine
great discomfort has been expressed at many levels about doctors
taking on a rationing role. Fundholding GPs have been recorded
as expressing misgivings, or outright opposition, to the taking on
of a rationing role (Ayres 1996). It has been argued that rationing
does not sit comfortably with the deontological element of medical ethics, the duty to the individual patient which makes very
difficult any trading off of benefit to one patient against benefit to
another (Smith and Morissey 1994). In social work the response
has been rather different. At the practice level it has been largely
accepted by social workers that limited resources must be used
to the best effect and that this means not everyone will get
everything that would be useful to them. It has also meant that

considerable ingenuity has been used to achieve the best mix, despite the constraints of management guidelines since the early 1990s (Leat and Perkins 1998). The social work critique of rationing emerges not at the level of professional ethics but at the political level. Social work as a profession has taken on a more radical political agenda than either nursing or medicine, in which under-resourcing of services is seen as a manifestation of an unjust and oppressive society.

Rationing is alien to the ethics of nursing as it is to those of the other two professions. The code of professional conduct says nothing about the fair distribution of resources, whereas it emphasises strongly the individual nurse's commitment to the well-being and autonomy of the individual patient. However, it is clear from the experience of the medical profession that it is quite possible to find oneself placed in a rationing role even where this is in conflict with ones perception of professional ethics. I would suggest that this is probably what is beginning to happen to the nursing profession. I would also suggest that this is a beneficial development for health care, for nursing, and for the new health consensus, and should be pursued positively. This development is located specifically in primary care, where community nurses are now represented on the board of primary care trusts. These bodies have a rationing function as predicted by Pickard and Sheaff (1999), and although there is not as yet a clear and public acknowledgment of this fact, it is implicit in their function, and is emerging in the developing analysis of their role as this takes shape. In a situation where there is a gap between patient need and demand on the one hand and availability on the other, such decisions will have to be made, and the powers delegated to PCTs means that it is they that will make the detailed decisions with regard to the prioritising of resources and the restriction of those provisions where demand exceeds supply. As with fundholding GPs there may be some discomfort about this development among board members, committee members and managers within PCTs. However, it is hard to see how it is to be avoided.

It is likely that nurses, as newcomers to rationing decisions, will initially be influenced by existing professional approaches to rationing. The models available to them in this situation are medical, managerial and economic. The medical approach is mainly concerned with individual rationing, and has in the past been either covert or engaged in unwillingly. In recent years there have been moves toward a more explicit medical approach (Crisp *et al.* 1997) though this departs somewhat from the traditional medical emphasis on duty to maximise benefit to the individual patient. The managerial approach focuses on prioritising rather than rationing, and is traditionally geared to maximising health gain. However, Ham and McIver (2000) suggest that for those prioritising at this level the way decisions are made is as important as the outcome, requiring rationality, openness and accountability. The economic model, underpinned by the discipline of health economics, focuses more narrowly on aspects of health gain and is best exemplified by the concept of QALYs (Quality Adjusted Life Years) as a means of measuring the health and other gains of specific interventions (Williams 1985).

None of these models is in itself sufficient to help professionals and managers to engage the public in a debate about rationing and prioritising. The medical model has not yet emerged sufficiently from a tradition of secrecy and denial to provide an effective basis, although medical thinking on rationing in recent years has a great deal to contribute. The managerial approach is helpful in emphasising the combining of rationality and openness, but the ideal of comprehensive rationality, wherein all data and all criteria are factored in, is, in the view of Klein *et al.* (1996), of doubtful realism. The economic model scores best on precision and rationality, but achieves this at the cost of being very narrow in focus. None of these provides an adequate model for nurses as they become involved in the process. There is a need for nursing to develop its own prioritising and rationing agenda, which will work within the spirit of nursing ethics, while at the same time extending the range of the ethical tradition of nursing to include what is at present excluded. In the next section I consider the kind of approach to rationing that would serve best in these respects.

Justice in prioritising and rationing

It is useful at this point to consider some general principles relevant to this process. First there are considerations of convenience and expediency. These will be different for all those involved, as it will depend entirely on their interests what kind of decisions are convenient and expedient for them. It is expedient for government to persuade the electorate that it is well served by public services despite low taxes, and government will only depart from that tightrope when an upsurge of public concern and agitation requires it to do so. Such an upsurges generally involve the media, whose interests lie in highlighting issues amenable to simplification, raising public concern and drawing readers/viewers accordingly. The professions have an interest in the development and resourcing of their specialist interests, and in the extension of their professional boundaries and powers, alongside the minimising of external interference, either from government or public. Government and managers, by contrast, will seek as much control and surveillance as possible over those actually delivering health care, while minimising the public responsibility which *they* carry for the less popular aspects of that delivery. The public, meanwhile, will seek to minimise as far as possible its tax burden, while at the same time worrying as little as possible about unpleasant topics such as illness and mortality. When aroused, however, the public will want a quick and accommodating response from government. All of these players operate according to political and social forces that lead them, quite rationally, in several different directions, and toward conflicting agendas. In this context there is no reason why the distribution of health care resources should approximate to any recognisable notion of fairness and justice, or why the interests of the most vulnerable of all participants – the patient – should be protected. This, I hope, offers a rationale as to why considerations of expediency and convenience do not provide a sufficient basis for rationing and prioritising in health care.

However, we need to make a case for considerations of justice and the protection of the vulnerable being included in the decision-making frame. I argued in Chapter 1 that health is a good which, though not itself a moral good, has some characteristics in common with a moral good. The ascription of health involves a mixture of description and evaluation and the full appreciation of health probably requires the development of a degree of cultivated awareness, as does the appreciation of beauty, wisdom and moral good. I also suggested that the valuation of health is not culturally specific, even though descriptions of health do vary somewhat culturally. For these reasons the distribution of health care resources is a matter of considerable importance. We are not simply dealing with the wherewithal for an efficient and prosperous society, as we might be if we were arguing about, for instance, the distribution of public or private transport. We are dealing with a fundamental human good. We know that health care is not the only, or even always the best means to optimise health. But it is the most important means that is explicitly and primarily geared to that purpose. We can reasonably demand that most of every pound spent on health will actually go toward the optimising of health. We would not expect this with housing, or education, despite their health benefits. So health care is special in the sense that it has a special relationship with a special good. It is also true that health is closely associated with two fundamental definitions of moral good – well-being in the utilitarian model and autonomy in the Kantian model. Health is fundamentally important for both of these. For all these reasons the distribution of health care re-sources is a matter that needs to be regulated by appropriate ethical principles, and not simply by considerations of political expediency or convenience. The moral framework for the distri-bution of goods among people is generally provided by the con-cept of distributive justice, and that is why these considerations have been identified by writers on this issue as necessary to pro-vide a framework for managing the conflicting agendas identified above. It is those considerations that I now discuss.

Distributive justice concerns the development of an ethical framework for the allocation of goods in society. As such, it takes account of several moral considerations that in normal moral dis-course we would see as relevant to questions of 'who gets what?'. These can be quickly recounted. First, we ought to give the re-source to those who need it most; second, we ought to give the resource to those who will benefit most from it; third, we ought to give the resource to those who are entitled to it/have a right to it; fourth we ought to give the resource to those who deserve it; and fifth, we ought to give the resource in a way that is equitable and will rectify existing inequality, or maintain existing equality.

Need
The concept of need as a basis for distributive priority seems at first sight to be ethically incontrovertible. To give most to those whose need is greatest seems on the face of it the securest moral basis for priority. However, the concept of need is itself problem-atic, and includes two elements that seem to pull in opposite

directions. Need for a treatment has often been defined as the ability to benefit from that treatment (Hurley *et al.* 1997). But this implies that the criterion is actually one of utility rather than need and that we should be providing treatment in a way that achieves the greatest possible benefit. This would suggest that the criteria of need and utility are in fact the same thing, so we can shorten our list of considerations from five to four. However, this does not exhaust the issue. Need does not consist solely of the ability to benefit. It also consists in normal usage of the severity of the problem that is being suffered by the potential recipient. My need is greater if my problem is more severe. Clearly we can only say this about need for a treatment that is relevant to the problem. If I am suffering acute liver failure, I have no need of a renal transplant, because it would do me no good. My need is for a liver transplant. And here the two aspects of need come into conflict. If I am suffering acute liver failure after a debilitating period of chronic liver failure my ability to benefit from the transplant may be diminished by my overall diminished state of health. So one facet of need, the severity of my condition, may compromise the other facet of need, my ability to benefit. On this basis I suggest that the concept of need is not in fact a unitary concept in this context, and must be seen as overlapping a good deal with utility.

Utility
The principle of using resources in order to achieve the most benefit is the essence of the utility principle, and its roots in utilitarianism are apparent. It is an application of the principle that in every instance our choice between options should be guided by the goal of maximising a specific good. The original utilitarians' chosen good was happiness or pleasure (Mill 1962), but well-being and health have both been recruited for the same purpose (Beauchamp and Childress 1994). However, they are not interchangeable. Our choice of good will determine our other choices. The link with utilitarianism also opens up a wider issue in relation to the principle of utility. In the discussion of need as a principle, I confined my consideration to the needs of the patient. But utilitarianism does not permit this limiting of focus. Utilitarianism requires us to maximise well-being generally, not to concentrate on the well-being of specified individuals. In the case of health care, that principle will not necessarily lead us toward

prioritising patients who are most likely to benefit from treatment, but rather to provide treatment where it is most likely to maximise well-being, which is quite a different matter. If, for instance we have a choice between patients with or without dependent families in the provision of a life-saving treatment, and we can ascertain that the families will benefit from the survival of the patient, it is likely that we should prioritise patients with dependent families, other things being equal. We could legitimately choose to treat a patient with a more dubious prognosis, on the basis that if that patient does recover, the number of people who benefit from that will be greater than in the case of a patient with a better prognosis but no family.

As Dickenson (1999) points out this means that the use of utilitarian principles to guide priorities leads us into territory that is at variance with proclaimed medical criteria. There is evidence that in some situations doctors will take account of the effects on family and others of their choices of prioritising treatment. For instance Crisp *et al.* (1997) include this as a legitimate consideration for a GP practice. But it remains controversial. Generally the patient's own prospect of benefiting from the treatment remains the central rationing criterion for the medical profession, and there are certainly arguments against taking account of family or others' benefit. One of these is a utilitarian argument; that taking account of the well-being of families and others would not work because it could not be done accurately. It would therefore fail to maximise well-being and would also lose credibility with the public. If we cannot overcome this difficulty we risk failing to maximise well-being *and* creating disbenefits by destroying public confidence in the health service. The other argument against taking account of potential benefit to families and dependents is a deontological or contractarian rather than a utilitarian argument. This runs to the effect that there is a special obligation on the part of health care personnel to attend to the well-being of those who are sick which does not extend to other people. This could be based on the concept of professional duty, which locates the professional obligation primarily with the patient. Or it could be based on the idea of an implicit contract between the health services and professionals on the one hand, and the public on the other hand, which includes that same obligation to prioritise those who are sick. Although the reality of health care is that it is not always possible to make a clear distinction between 'patient' and 'others', in most situations where individual rationing is necessary, that distinction is reasonably clear.

Another problem of utilitarianism is that it places no requirement on us to favour the worst-off in our maximising of well-being. In seeking to improve someone's health, the level from which that person is starting is not part of the equation, only the distance they travel. In this respect the utility principle contrasts starkly with the need-as-severity-of-illness principle, and reveals another problem for the utilitarian approach. In situations where the most ill, and most disadvantaged, are more expensive to help than the less ill and the more advantaged, the latter will always be prioritised. In practice that applies not only to the debilitated acute liver failure patient whose prospect of benefiting from a transplant are less than those of a fitter patient. It also applies to the disadvantaged housing estate where a large input of health promotion money is needed to reduce levels of drug dependency, teenage pregnancy and cardiovascular problems. On a neighbouring estate with more limited problems, where there is already a better infrastructure of community resources, more could be achieved with less money. Our reasons for favouring the sickest and the worst-off need therefore to be rooted in a different principle.

Equality
One basis for caring for the sickest might be the principle of care, enjoining us to respond to suffering. This provides a basis for the prioritising of the worst-off and seeing them as in greatest need. The other counterbalancing principle to the rational priorities of utilitarianism is the third of the principles of distributive justice, that of equality. The equitable distribution of health care resources to minimise inequality and maximise equality is rooted in the notion of human equality of worth, which owes a good deal to the Kantian idea of the moral specialness of the person. Kant's view that persons belong to a special category and carry a special moral value implies that all persons are in that particular sense of equally special moral value (Paton 1978). That value is compromised if there is avoidable inequality in health, because health is necessary for survival and autonomy, which are in turn necessary concomitants for personhood. It is therefore morally justified,

even imperative, to seek to promote equality in terms of health and health care.

However, the concept of equality must apply to something specific. In which *ways* ought people to be equal? Different ways of being equal do not always coexist well. In broader social and political terms welfare states struggle with the choice between equality of opportunity and equality of outcome, knowing that the former will not lead to the latter. In terms of health care there is an equivalent issue between equality of access to health care according to need (often referred to as equity) and equality of health. Equity will not necessarily produce equality of health because people make different degrees of use of their access, and health care is not always equally effective, because of other differences. The problem with equity, probably the more achievable of the two outcomes, is that it is dependent on agreeing a concept of need, which leads us back into our problems with the definition of need. If need is ability to benefit, then equity would justify prioritising those more likely to benefit, often those who are less ill. Full equality of health is probably impossible to achieve through health care alone, which may in fact not be always the most effective way of pursuing it (Arblaster *et al.* 1996). But this does not invalidate attempts to move toward equality, as an expression of the fundamental Kantian principles of human worth. And that fundamental justification certainly provides an argument for ensuring that our actions never exacerbate existing inequalities. It is in this area that the principle of equality counterbalances the principle of utility.

Rights

The fourth principle of distributive justice, rights, is similar to the principle of need in that it impinges on the argument in two very different ways, in accordance with a distinction made by Miller (1976). Miller divides rights into two kinds; positive rights, which are contingent on a particular system of provision, and only have meaning in that context; and ideal rights, which have an absolute status, standing above particular social or legal provisions. This represents the difference between rights to a particular benefit in a particular system and what are sometimes referred to as basic human rights, such as those set out in the United Nations Declaration (UN 1948). In terms of positive rights, that is, the rights provided for within a particular system of health care, the individual's right to health care depends on their status within that system in the country where they are located. In the UK the NHS provides health care free at the point of use to all residents, and this can be interpreted as a right, insofar as the resident can claim an entitlement to health care. In the US the individual right to health care is dependent on their relationship to a particular health care system. If I subscribe to a particular health insurance scheme I have a right to the health care available within that insurance scheme. In a universal system like that of the UK the problem with the concept of a positive right is that where resources are limited, that right is inevitably compromised. The fact that all citizens have an equal right makes it impossible to use the concept of rights in a positive way to prioritise or ration, though it provides an argument against disadvantaging any group or individual.

The other category of rights, ideal rights, work differently. We ascribe such rights to people irrespective of whether or not their governments recognise and respect such rights, and regard them as fundamental to being human. We might argue that people have a basic human right to free health care even in a country where no health service exists. We may use such an argument to advocate the provision of health care in that country. However, again the concept does not seem to help us in situations of prioritising and rationing, because the basic human right to health care, if we believe it to exist, must be universal to all persons. Essentially the concept of right can only be used to argue against depriving some people of treatment but not others, or to argue in favour of a greater proportion of the national stock of resources to be devoted to health care, to a point where rationing becomes unnecessary.

Desert
The final principle in my list is that of desert. This largely applies to rationing choices between individual and rests on the question: does this person deserve treatment? We generally understand the idea of deserving something to be based on merit. Getting what we deserve recognises and rewards a level of moral merit and conversely, to be defined as not deserving of something is seen as the response to moral failure or turpitude. In terms of health care the idea of deserving has been introduced into situations where individuals can be seen as having deliberately or negligently

damaged their health and have therefore lost a position of deservingness in relation to health care. The argument arises as to whether smokers are less deserving of heart bypass operations than non-smokers (Underwood and Bailey 1993). The same argument arises with alcoholics in relation to liver transplants (Moss and Siegler 1991). The problem with using desert as a principle of rationing is that we are using health care as a reward, and its withholding (or at least delaying) as a punishment. In this sense we are using it as an equivalent to the award of an OBE, or being fined. It is fairly clear that health care is not suitable for this kind of use. Our health care system was created to respond to a universal human need, and is ultimately concerned with the individual's prospects of survival. None of the recognised rewards and punishments that we regard as legitimate in our society is of this type, and it makes no moral sense to use health care in that way.

Nurses and distributive justice

The most useful principles in the above deliberation seem to be utility and equality. Each balances the other, and between them they absorb the concept of need, at least in moral terms. The concept of rights has largely negative relevance to the business of prioritising and rationing, much of which is absorbed by the principle of equality. The concept of desert seems inappropriate in this frame. So how do these relate to the nursing profession and its discomfort with the whole rationing issue? If nurses are to engage the public in a process of debate and education moving toward a consensus on health, can they include the issues of rationing and prioritising in this, when the profession seems very uncertain of its own position? If we start from what we know about nursing, about its ethics and the priorities of its members, we can start to come to a view on this. Nursing ethics focus on the well-being of the patient, both in terms of their care and in terms of their dignity and autonomy. The nursing approach tends to be individualistic, and nurses on the whole are not given to thinking in collective terms (Browne 2001). In this they are to some degree like doctors, though the medical profession on the whole has moved some way toward taking account of collective issues. They are unlike social workers, who tend to operate in a collective and contextual framework.

However, the nursing profession has the potential to develop a distinctive perspective on rationing and prioritising. The nursing emphasis on patient uniqueness, paradoxically, provides a strong basis for the equal treatment of patients. This, combined with the ethical principle of care, provides a counterbalance to the established primacy of the utilitarian view. That is the key to the nursing position on rationing and prioritising. I described earlier what I termed the medical, the managerial and the health economics models of prioritising and rationing. All of these in different ways emphasise the patient's ability to benefit from treatment and the effectiveness of treatment in guiding decisions about priorities. The medical model sees this in individual terms, and the other models in collective terms, but the essential view remains the same. In terms of rationality the arguments in favour of maximising benefit are powerful and a rationally managed NHS needs to be strongly influenced by this. However, it only represents one of what I have argued to be two key principles in rationing and prioritising. The principle of equality, applied to severity of need, enables us to balance the utilitarian fear of wasting resources on the more ill and more disadvantaged with a principle of equality of worth for those less productive patients, and of equality of care for those who are very sick. This principle offers the basis for a nursing model of resource allocation to balance the medical, managerial and economic models. It applies both at the individual level and at the collective, community level. At the individual level the principle of equality chimes in with the values of the nursing profession and at the collective level it chimes in also with the policy direction of the present government. As the government's stated commitment to reduce health inequalities is accompanied by an expressed desire to involve the nursing profession in this process (Department of Health 1999) there is potential for a synergy between nursing values and the expressed values underpinning this policy.

In order to influence the rationing and prioritising agenda, I would suggest a dual strategy for nursing. First, nurses need to develop their involvement with decision-making at the levels where prioritising and rationing decisions are made. Nurses are already involved in their own right in PCT boards and subcommittees, and as managers in the health authority level of decision-making. The next step is to ensure that nursing's particular contribution to the processes of rationing and prioritising is fully realised and optimised. I have outlined what I think the basis of this contribution is. What remains is for it to be articulated and developed in decision-making arenas. This needs to manifest not only in the content of discussion at PCT boards and committees, but also in a wider agenda of encouraging openness within the system in discussing rationing and prioritising issues.

This is one part of a dual strategy. The other part points in a different direction toward the public and the patient. I have argued in earlier chapters that nurses have a particular combination of skills and characteristics that enable them to form a vital link between the health care system and the public. These include communication skills tuned particularly to the business of acting as interpreter between the patient and the rest of the health care system. They also include an ability to focus on process as well as outcome. I have suggested that these skills need to be tuned to working with the public and the patient toward a new articulated consensus on health. A central part of that process will inevitably focus on rationing and prioritising, and again the activities of health promotion offer a vehicle for a process of exploration and education of the public in these areas. At present, what relatively limited evidence exists suggests a significant gap between the public's choices of health priority groups as against the professional's choices (Bowling 1996). Given the complexity of the area and the fact that differing priorities can be supported by equally valid arguments, it is doubtful whether it would be possible or desirable to seek to remove those differences. Our goal is not a fully congruent consensus but rather an articulated consensus where holders of different positions are aware of points of connection with other positions and value these sufficiently to sustain a sense of common commitment to health as a good. It is particularly important that that articulation is achieved in relation to rationing and prioritising, where a failure to understand and appreciate other positions might lead to injustice and exclusion of a fundamental kind. It is vital therefore that a dialogue between the public and the health care system includes this area.

At present the public's perceptions are partly formed by what we might see as concerns that are psychologically and morally coherent, for instance a desire to prioritise the health of children. Other public priorities may be based on simple lack of information about the effectiveness of particular kinds of health care. According to Bowling (1996) the public are relatively uninterested in community care, and are very interested in acute care. At present as Richardson and Waddington (1996) point out, their preferences are also influenced by the media's agenda, which is inevitably biased toward the more dramatic and individualised kinds of health care. They may to some degree be influenced by the politicians' agenda (mediated through the media), and it is not clear that an honest debate on health care priorities is always in the politicians' interests. So, the public carry a burden of misinformation alongside their own valid perceptions. Therefore a careful balance has to be achieved between informing, educating and clarifying misconceptions on the one hand, and respecting the integrity of the citizen's priorities on the other hand. This process of informing and clarifying, but also listening and respecting, is one that is central to the nurse's repertoire and which nurses can reasonably expect to do effectively. Already they do it effectively in relation to many aspects of patient care. The extra element that is required here is a clear and confident nursing perspective on these issues, not to be imposed on the patient, but to provide the basis for the nurse to engage the citizen in a debate on the issue.

Conclusion

Public legitimacy in health care is nowhere more important than in the area of rationing and resource allocation decisions. Where the public sees such decisions as unjust, either in terms of outcome or in terms of process, this erodes the trust between citizen and health care system, in a situation where that bond is already somewhat delicate. Nursing can offer a perspective on this issue, which forms a bridge between the somewhat single-track perspectives of other influential groups, and the more diffuse responses of the public. It is a key area for nursing to facilitate the dialogue toward articulated consensus.

10 Nurses and organisational learning

Introduction

This chapter focuses on the nurse's relationship with the organisations that deliver health care, and that in many cases also perform the role of employer to the individual nurse. Organisations have already had some consideration in Chapter 5, but the particular purpose here is to link organisational considerations more explicitly to the business of working for an articulated consensus, and also to consider the issues arising for nurses, and possible ways forward for nursing, where conflicts of loyalty arise between the nurse and the organisation.

Learning organisations

I have argued from Chapter 7 onward that nursing as a profession has a particular role to play in promoting and facilitating a debate on health and health care moving toward a new kind of consensus on health. This leads us into an additional dimension in our analysis of the problem of the nurse in relation to her employing organisation. Put simply, if the case for dialogue and debate is to be made, and if it is to prevail, this needs to happen through the organisation's own machinery. I would extend this point somewhat further, to suggest that that debate needs also to happen within the organisation. The need for an articulated consensus on health and health care requires that those working within the machinery of health care are part of the articulation, alongside the public they serve. This requires a culture of open and critical debate within the organisation and it also requires the organisation to corporately contribute to the development of articulated consensus. This in turn requires that the organisation has certain characteristics. These characteristics relate to what is sometimes termed the 'learning organisation' (Senge 1994). This is an organisation with sufficient self-awareness to identify limiting and sub-optimal patterns within its practices and procedures; and, more importantly to be able to identify and remedy within itself defensive forms of communication and information-management that perpetuate those sub-optimal practices. There is much evidence that organisations tend to develop defensive patterns that censor out challenging or problematic information, and develop instead an investment in maintaining existing perceptions and practices. It is these that are in the frame.

It is not an easy matter to develop a culture within an organisation that is fully alert to all relevant information from within as well as outside, and also able to debate and interpret that information in an open way. Several writers have devoted a good deal of thought to ways in which organisations can become 'learning organisations' (Argyris and Schon 1978; March 1999). The additional responsibilities of clinical governance mean in any case that this is an imperative for organisations such as NHS trusts. But for trusts to open themselves to debate with the outside world about the nature of health and health care requires that they have the capacity to also debate internally, and to be able to live with uncertainty about fundamental definitions.

In some ways the groundwork for the learning organisation has been laid in the NHS since the 1980s, in the form of quality assurance mechanisms. The concept of quality assurance involves building in a feedback loop that provides one of the basic components of a learning organisation (Ellis and Whittington 1993) and the last two decades have seen that loop become increasingly sophisticated and comprehensive, contributing to the change in relationship between organisation and professions. The development of clinical governance as part of the post-1997 wave of NHS reforms sought to make the learning process more inclusive by placing a clearer and heavier responsibility for the maintenance of professional standards of practice upon the organisations delivering health care, particularly trusts (Buetow and Roland 1999). To respond to this requirement, trusts have set up machinery to monitor and improve professional standards and to respond to deficits in those standards. Among other developments, this has led to a rapid development of machinery for ethical scrutiny (for instance clinical ethics committees) operating often in an advisory role, with a close relationship to clinical governance (Slowther *et al.* 2001). That development in itself is indicative of how much of the traditional professional agenda has now become the concern of the organisation. In the past the formal consideration of ethical issues was largely the preserve of the professional bodies whose task it has been to develop codes of ethics and to respond to unethical behaviour on the part of professionals. At the time of writing, it seems unlikely that trust ethics committees will usurp the latter function in the near future, but the formulation of trust codes of conduct seems to be an identifiable focus of interest and activity within such bodies. Questions of duty, priority, utility and autonomy will also be part of the agenda of clinical ethics committees. And such deliberations will also lead them to a deeper consideration of the functions and policies of the trust itself – a development commended by Doyal (2001).

The implications of this development are not yet fully apparent, but it is possible to make a number of informed guesses about the way in which things may move. The distinction between professional considerations and professional duties on the one hand, and the requirements of employers on the other, is likely to become blurred. Issues of professional competence and professional duty (including the ethical dimension of that latter concept) will become matters which trusts, and trust management will increasingly feel both required to and competent to address. Historically, the assumption has been that the professional body is the guardian and guarantor of the professional's duty to the patient (and by virtue of that, guardian of the patient's interests) while the trust is concerned with the practical, technical business of organising the delivery of care, without the ethical discipline of the professional. But organisations can no longer be seen as ethically 'innocent', driven purely by the demands and constraints of their constituency and their environment. They will increasingly treat ethical issues as part of their concern. And the kind of ethical conflicts that have taken place between organisational and professional imperatives will take place to a far greater degree *within* the organisation. The machinery of clinical governance will provide the forum for at least some of those conflicts to be pursued.

The role of nurses in this process is likely to be central, for some of the same reasons that I have argued that nurses can play a central role in involving the public in debate. In particular, the combination of numerical strength and importance, clinical knowledge and communication skills that nurses bring to the debate means that they are most likely to be able to achieve a 'critical mass' through which cultural shift is possible. In the organisational context, however, there are other attributes that nurses bring to the situation. The knowledge base of nursing is particularly well geared to a situation of uncertainty in terms of definitions and goals. Nursing has a tradition of epistemological openness and focus which equips nurses to work with ideas that are fundamentally problematic and uncertain, while at the same time maintaining a pragmatic focus on practical usefulness (see, for instance, Stevenson and Beech 2001). In a context of uncertainty that is a great strength. The challenge for nurses will be to find the balance between sustaining an open debate within the organisation, and at the same time keeping some focus on the organisational politics that will inevitably accompany the process. The latter activity is a necessary concomitant to any major organisational development, as political skills will certainly be used by some protagonists, and therefore they must be used by all protagonists, to avoid an unjust imbalance of power. It is probably in this area that nurses need to become more practiced and confident if they are to make full use of their pivotal position in the health care system.

Nurses who are also senior managers have a particular role in this situation, although at first sight their position would seem to be a difficult one. The culture and traditions of nursing are strongly focused on individual patient care, and this distances the senior manager somewhat from their professional roots. The senior manager's main concern is less with patients as individuals and more with patients as a category. And the individualised nature of nursing ethics means that it is a good deal more difficult to draw clear guidance from the ethics and culture of the profession in terms of patients en masse than it is for patients as individuals. On the one hand, senior managers have more power than nurses lower in the hierarchy, so their decisions will affect more people, including nurses, other workers, and patients. On the other hand, it would be unusual for the decision of a senior manager to have the depth of impact on the life and well-being of an individual patient that the decision of a nurse working directly with that patient might have. For the manager the individual experience of health will be somewhat mediated by the business of maximising health for a population of patients, a process which will inevitably lead to a more quantitative, and less qualitative perspective on health. This in turn lends itself to a less care-centred and more utilitarian approach to the goals of health care. This perspective distances the senior manager from her professional ethical roots, and this has been seen by some commentators in negative terms, as marginalising nurse senior managers, cutting them off from their profession and trapping them in a non-nursing managerial culture (Fedoruk and Pincombe 2000).

However, from a professional point of view a commitment to maximising well-being within a population is every bit as valid as a commitment to providing optimum care for an individual patient. I would argue that the senior manager has a crucial role to play in connecting the utilitarian and the care-based perspectives of nursing in a way that allows nurses to interrogate their own perspectives on health. As an example, one of the more creative aspects of applying a utilitarian approach to health issues is that it requires one to quantitatively compare goods that are qualitatively different; to compare life expectancy with quality of life, or to compare alertness and autonomy with freedom from pain. This exercise requires a particularly focused consideration of the nature of health as a good, and its relationship to other goods. The risk is that it becomes a somewhat theoretical debate if it is not imbued with practice experience of different health states in patients. Those who can undertake this exercise most effectively are those with experience at both levels, of individual patient experience of different states of health and well-being, and also of resource management and prioritising at a senior level. This is where the nurse-senior manager has a particular contribution to make to the wider debate on health.

Conflicts with the organisation

Despite all of the above, there is a fair likelihood that conflicts will continue to arise between professional and organisational agendas, and that individuals and small groups of professionals will find themselves at odds with the methods and practices of the organisations within which they work. In a situation where debate and diversity is central to the conduct of health care, not every divergence of view will be satisfactorily resolved. In any case we cannot be sure that the machinery of clinical governance will actually optimise organisational learning, or successfully encompass the requirements of organisational and professional governance. It is clear from Argyris and Schon (1978), from Senge (1994) and from March (1999), that it is no simple matter for organisations to achieve optimal learning, and that rigidities and resistance often creep in. In particular, we cannot be sure that the range of feedback that the machinery of clinical governance is able and willing to receive is sufficiently diverse. If the learning loop is too exclusive, the danger is that it will have the effect of reinforcing the organisation's certainty that it is functioning appropriately.

We need to consider what the nurse should do if she finds herself at odds with the practices of the organisation. Is it appropriate to wait and hope indefinitely for things to shift sufficiently to allow her to pursue the professional agenda with patients and community? If the nurse has used all her skills and knowledge to work for internal change and this is not happening, a different approach needs to be considered. Organisations are not ends in themselves but are means to an end. It they are not fulfilling their purpose and cannot be induced to do so through internal discussion, there is clearly an argument for drawing a deadline, beyond which the organisation is ignored, circumvented or opposed. There are many situations in which the professional freedom of the nurse may conflict with the employer's agenda. It may conflict over the effectiveness of particular health care provisions, the appropriateness of particular priorities, the truthfulness or helpfulness of particular messages given to the public by health care providers. In all these areas the professional agenda of the nurse may come into conflict with the agenda of the employer, and we need an ethical framework to consider this.

I propose to explore this by drawing on analogous considerations relating to the issue of whistle-blowing. The whistle-blower is normally understood as an employee who exposes poor practice or corrupt practice within their organisation. Such exposure may be geared to the public arena, or it may be directed toward a regulatory body. A number of cases have received publicity over recent years, usually because the individual who blew the whistle was subjected to reprisals by the organisation that was exposed (e.g. Pilgrim 1995). Even after the passing of the Public Interest Disclosure Act (Stationary Office 1998), which was intended to provide some protection for whistle-blowers, it appears that embarrassed employers can still find ways of punishing the whistle-blower.

The nurse's role in promoting debate on health care will not in most cases involve the kind of exposure and embarrassment of health care providers that whistle-blowers inflict. That may happen on occasions, but on the whole the most difficult aspect of the role involves the nurse seeing herself as free to criticise, and to deviate from any 'party line' that the provider might seek to impose. Crucially, the practical goal of whistle-blowing, to stop abuses and poor practice, is not necessarily going to have any part in the nurse's role in promoting debate. Also, the use of information to force a particular outcome goes against the spirit of open debate. So in that sense we are dealing with a different process from that of whistle-blowing. But in other ways there are significant similarities. The nurse who questions the practice or policies of her employer outside of the confines of the organisation may find that she is exposing the employer to media scrutiny, even if that is not her intention. Such an outcome would not necessarily be under her control. In that way her actions would compromise an asset which modern corporate bodies value highly, a consistent and positive corporate image. In that respect the nurse is in a similar position to the whistle-blower. It is therefore worth considering the kind of arguments that seem relevant, in order to provide an ethical framework for nurses to work within.

The first question that the critical nurse needs to ask is a utilitarian one – is her action going to do more good than harm overall? The same question is relevant to whistle-blowing, and it is true that the whistle-blower may indeed do significant harm through the disruption and loss of reputation suffered by an organisation that might on balance still be performing a beneficial role despite specific weaknesses. In the case of whistle-blowing, abuses may be of such an order that once exposed, providers feel constrained to act dramatically to remedy those abuses. Such actions may be hurried and ill-considered and motivated as much by issues of public and media images as by a desire to rectify short-comings. They are therefore likely to be deleterious to services. A good example of this is the case of Ashworth hospital, where an oppressive, excessively punitive regime was exposed, creating a considerable scandal. The hospital authorities overreacted and created a situation where abuses of the opposite kind – members of the public, including children being put at risk through an over-lax regime – then occurred. These were exposed in turn, with a high level of publicity (Donnelly 1999). It seems clear in this case that the initial act of whistle-blowing did not lead to an improvement of services but achieved the opposite result. From a utilitarian viewpoint it was therefore not justified.

The critical nurse is less likely to do significant harm unless she triggers an extreme and disruptive response in the employer. The measured querying of a provider's assumptions and (perhaps) policies and practices in terms of models and goals of health should not provoke such an extreme reaction, because by their nature the issues being raised are matters of legitimate debate, and their broaching need not be a matter of embarrassment or discredit for the provider. The only potential embarrassment arises, as I suggested, from having an employee who questions these things. It is doubtful, however, whether the impact of this process on a provider's corporate image is likely to lead to real harm to services or to patients. The corporate image is essentially an instrument of information control and manipulation, and its implications for patient services are probably best seen as neutral. The provider may nonetheless overreact to this, which may well be a problem for the nurse. So the calculation of harm as against gain would be very different from the nurse who simply raises questions as against the nurse who blows the whistle. The main issue is probably going to concern her relationship with her employer and the effect on her career. This is clearly a significant matter.

The other question is one of loyalty and duty. There is a sense in which employees have a duty to their employer, based on the contract of employment and perhaps on other obligations entered into. Whether this is a moral duty is open to debate, but from a Kantian point of view the contract of employment can be taken as involving a promise on the employee's part (and likewise on the employer's part) which may then have moral force on the basis of the categorical imperative to keep promises. On the other hand the nurse also has a duty to the patient. This is arguably also based on a promise, though not a direct one. My argument for this is as follows. By registering with the NMC, each nurse commits herself to the code of professional conduct, which constitutes a public promise to behave in certain ways. That promise is made to the public, which includes each patient who encounters each nurse. Clearly most patients will not have read the code of conduct, or indeed have heard of the NMC, but the declaration is nonetheless publicly made, and that is sufficient to constitute a promise.

In the whistle-blowing situation the nurse's conflict is often between duty to employer and duty to patient and it has been argued that the duty to the patient should normally take precedence (Wilmot 2001). This is because the employer is an organisation, while the patient is a person. The argument runs to the effect that organisations, whilst having some of the characteristics of persons (they can make decisions, and perhaps can be held responsible for those decisions) do not have the moral status of persons because they are not ends in themselves. Every organisation was created for a purpose, and its existence is limited by that purpose. In this, organisations are quite different from, and morally inferior to persons, who exist as ends in themselves and have no need of a purpose outside of themselves. Although persons may choose to commit themselves to a specific purpose, this is an expression of their autonomy, and they can equally easily abandon that purpose without compromising their moral status. Because Kant never considered the moral status of organisations, I cannot argue that he regarded promises to organisations as inferior to promises to persons. But one of the consequences of breaking a promise is that we treat the promisee as a means rather than an end. We are using a linguistic form to manipulate another person to our ends. The Kantian categorical imperative requires that persons must always be treated as ends, and this gives persons primacy over organisations in relation to promise-keeping (Paton 1978). My argument therefore is that in a case of conflict, we should (other things being equal) break our promise to an organisation rather than a person, and this gives the patient priority over the organisation.

This, again, provides a clearer guide in the case of whistle-blowing than it does in the case of the critical nurse questioning policy or practice. This is for the opposite reason from that cited in the case of the utilitarian consideration of harm. In that case

I suggested that the organisation's performance (and therefore patients) are unlikely to be harmed by questioning. In this case however, it would make more sense to say that individual patients are unlikely to derive clear and measurable benefit from the nurse's activity in engaging them in a critical dialogue. The benefits of dialogue are subtle, long-term, cumulative and dispersed, rather than clear, immediate and individual. The gains of the dialogue are for the community as a whole and for the overall benefit that they can derive from an appropriate health care system. So if the provider argues that the critical nurse is in breach of her contract, it is more difficult for the nurse to argue that she is adhering to a more pressing duty, that to the patient. There is nothing in the code of conduct that can be unambiguously construed as a promise to engage in the kind of dialogue that I am suggesting. So if the employer is able to argue effectively that such action is in breach of the promise implied by the contract of employment, this will be difficult to counter.

However, there *is* a counter to that argument, which is based on the nature of the provider organisation, and in particular its moral status as a non-person existing for a specific purpose. I argued earlier that organisations must have a purpose – that organisations are in essence patterns of co-operative behaviour by human beings, and that all co-operative behaviour between humans has a purpose. That purpose may be mutual enjoyment of one another's company, or the manufacture of cars, or the provision of health care. Whoever sets up the organisation and decides its purpose legitimises its existence. In some kinds of organisation, such as voluntary groups, the membership sets it up and defines its purpose. In the case of commercial companies those who invest in the creation and continuation of the company, the owners or shareholders, define its purpose. The management and employees of a company cannot change the purpose of that company of their own volition. This can only be done with the agreement of the shareholders. In the case of a NHS trust the bodies that set it up and confer its legitimacy on it are, primarily, central government. In each of these three cases of different types of organisations, the people or organisations that created and legitimised their existence have been termed the organisations constituency (Wilmot 1997). The organisation can be seen as being accountable to its constituency at a fundamental level. It exists and has its purpose, only by the will of the constituency. In the context of the British NHS most organisations have been created through legislation, and express the intention of that legislation. Changes or elaborations of their purpose emanate from government.

The agenda of central government in relation to health is to optimise the health of the population, while preventing health care resources from encroaching on the resources for other goods. This principle was pursued by the conservative governments of the 1980s and the '90s in a way that emphasised the responsibility of the individual (Department of Health 1992). The present Labour government has sought to take a different approach, with more emphasis on community responsibility and solidarity (Department of Health 1999). The case that I have put forward throughout this book is that the development of a modern health care system appropriate to contemporary society requires the development of a new kind of consensus on health, for which I have used the term articulated consensus. Whether we follow a more individualised approach in the Thatcherite tradition, or a partially communitarian approach in accordance with New Labour's agenda, that kind of consensus is, I would argue, a basic requirement. Insofar as it is part of the government agenda to will the end, then they must also will the means. So movement toward such a consensus must become part of the purpose of government policy, and therefore of the purpose of the organisations whose function it is to carry out that policy. Traditional approaches to the involvement of the public and the patient, assuming acceptance of established conceptions of health and health care, will not help to achieve those goals. This needs to be pursued through the kind of dialogue that I have been advocating throughout the last four chapters. Health provider organisations that discourage or prevent the pursuit of that dialogue are in effect obstructing the pursuit of a clearly established and acknowledged government purpose in health. In that sense they are working against the purpose of their existence that is defined and legitimised by government. The management of such an organisation has no right to use the resources of that organisation toward a purpose that conflicts with the organisation's legitimate purpose. They are in a real sense misusing those resources.

An organisation can only claim the commitment of its employees to work for its legitimate purposes. No contract of employment can legitimately require anything else. Not only can an employee legitimately claim that they have no duty to work for purposes outside those legitimate purposes. They can also claim that they should in fact be working for those legitimate purposes even where this conflicts with the practices of the existing management. Their duty as employee does not change simply because a particular management has its own illegitimate agenda. For nurses it is also necessary that their employer's legitimate agenda is in accord with their professional duty. However, as I said above, the code of professional conduct is not specific enough on the issue to allow us to argue that nurses have a professional duty to pursue the debate on health. In order for that to become part of the contract between the state and the nursing profession, the case must be made and both parties convinced that that is the appropriate direction for nursing to go. The creation of the Nursing and Midwifery Council, and the formulation of a new code of conduct (NMC 2002) have created a historic opportunity for this renegotiation.

Conclusion

In a situation where policy shifts are frequent, and manifestations of policy often ambiguous, the organisations delivering health care operate in an unstable and sometimes murky environment. They are frequently subject of contradictory pressure, from both within and outside, and it is not surprising that their behaviour is sometimes erratic. Nurses, as stakeholders in the health care system, have good reason to fight for their vision of the health care process at the organisational level as well as at the national level. A robust, critical approach to organisational behaviour by nurses could make a significant contribution, in the long run, to the building of a deeper trust between the public and the health care system.

References

Allmark, P. (1995) Can there be an ethics of care? *Journal of Medical Ethics*, **21**(1), 19–24.

Anderson, R., Aaronson, N. and Wilkin, D. (1993) A critical review of the international assessments of health-related quality of life, *Quality of Life Research*, **2**(4), 369–95.

Arblaster, L., Lambert, M., Entwhistle, V., Forster, M., Fullerton, D., Shelton, T. and Watt, I. (1996) A systematic review of the effectiveness of health service interventions aimed at reducing inequalities in health, *Journal of Health Service Research and Policy*, **1**(2), 93–103.

Argyris, C. and Schon, D. (1978) *Organisational Learning*. London: Addison-Wesley.

Ayres, P. (1996) Rationing health care: views from general practice, *Social Science and Medicine*, **42**(7), 1021–25.

Bain, J. (1994) Fundholding: a two tier system? *British Medical Journal*, **309**, 396–9.

Baker, M. (2000) *Making Sense of the White Papers*. Abingdon: Radcliffe.

Barlow, A. and Duncan, S. (2000) New Labour's communitarianism, supporting families and the 'rationality' mistake, Part 2, *Journal of Social Welfare and Family Law*, **22**(2), 129–44.

Bartlett, W. and LeGrand, J. (1994) The performance of trusts, in R. Robinson and J. LeGrand (eds), *Evaluating the NHS Reforms*. London: King's Fund. pp. 54–73.

Beattie, A. (1995) War and peace among the health tribes, in K. Soothill, L. Mackay and C. Webb (eds), *Interprofessional Relations in Health Care*. London: Edward Arnold, pp. 11–26.

Beauchamp, T. and Childress, J. (1994) *The Principles of Biomedical Ethics*, 4th edn. New York: Oxford University Press.

Beck, U. (1992) *Risk Society: toward a new modernity*. London: Sage.

Benner, P. and Wrubel, J. (1989) *The Primacy of Caring: Stress and coping in health and illness*. Menlo Park CA: Addison-Wesley.

Bentham, J. (1962) Introduction to the Principles of Morals and Legislation, in M. Warnock (ed.), *Utilitarianism*. London: Collins.

Biestek, F. (1957) *The Casework Relationship*. Chicago: Loyola University Press.

Blane, D. (1997) Health Professions, in G. Scambler (ed.), *Sociology as Applied to Medicine*. London: Saunders, pp. 212–24.

Blaxter, M. (1987) Self-reported health, in B. Cox, M. Blaxter, A. Bucke *et al.* (eds), *The Health and Lifestyle Survey*. London: Health Promotion Research Trust, 5–16.

Bordo, S. (1993) *Unbearable weight: feminism, western culture and the body*. Berkeley CA: University of California Press.

Bowling, A. (1996) Health care rationing: the public's debate, *British Medical Journal*, **312**: 670–4.

Bowling, A. (1998) *Measuring Health: a review of quality of life measurement scales.* Buckingham: Open University Press.

British Association of Social Workers (2002) *The Code of Ethics for Social Work.* Birmingham: BASW.

Browne, A. (2001) The influence of liberal political ideology on nursing science, *Nursing Inquiry,* **8**(2), 118–29.

Buetow, S. and Roland, M. (1999) Clinical Governance: bridging the gap between managerial and clinical approaches to quality of care, *Quality in Health Care,* **8**(3), 184–90.

Bunton, R. and Burrows, R. (1995) Consumption and Health in the epidemiological clinic of late modern medicine, in R. Bunton, S. Nettleton and R. Burrows (eds), *The Sociology of Health Promotion: Critical Analysis of Consumption, Lifestyle and Risk.* London: Routledge.

Bunton, R., Nettleton, S., and Burrows, R. (eds) (1995) *The Sociology of Health Promotion: Critical Analysis of Consumption, Lifestyle and Risk.* London: Routledge.

Bywaters, P. and McLeod, E. (2001) The impact of new labour's health policy on social services: a new deal for service users health? *British Journal of Social Work,* **31**(4), 579–94.

Carvel, J. (2001) Minority groups grow by 15%, *Guardian Newspaper,* 22 September 2001.

Central Council for Education and Training in Social Work (1991) *Rules and Requirements for the Diploma in Social Work* (Paper 30). London: CCETSW.

Chadwick, R. and Tadd, W. (1992) *Ethics and Nursing Practice.* Basingstoke: Macmillan – now Palgrave Macmillan.

Commission on Social Justice (1994) *Social Justice: strategies for national renewal.* London: Vintage.

Court, C. (1995) Survey shows widespread rationing in NHS, *British Medical Journal,* **311**, 1453–4.

Crisp, R., Hope, T. and Ebbs, D. (1997) The Asbury Draft Policy on Ethical Use of Resources, in B. New (ed.), *Rationing Talk and Action.* London: King's Fund.

Cronin, J.E. (1991) *The Politics of State Expansion.* London: Routledge.

Crossley, M. (2001a) 'Resistance' and health promotion, *Health Education Journal,* **60**(3), 197–204.

Crossley, M. (2001b) Rethinking psychological approaches towards health promotion, *Psychology and Health,* **16**(2), 161–77.

Cusveller, B. (1998) Cut from the right wood: spiritual and ethical pluralism in professional nursing practice, *Journal of Advanced Nursing,* **28**(2), 266–73.

Dalley, G. (1993) Professional ideology or organisational tribalism? The health service-social work divide, in J. Walmesley, J. Reynolds, P. Shakespeare and R. Woolfe (eds), *Health, Welfare and Practice.* London: Sage.

Daniels, N. (1985) *Just Health Care.* New York: Cambridge University Press.

Davies, C. (1995) *Gender and the Professional Predicament in Nursing.* Buckingham: Open University Press.

1. (1999) Falling public trust in health services: implications for untability, *Journal of Health Service Research and Policy*, **4**(4), 193–5.

.es, P. (2000) *Long-Term Care*. London: Mintel.

.geling, P., Hill, M., Kennedy, J., Coyle, B. and Maxwell, S. (2000) A cross-national study of differences in the identities of nursing in England and Australia, and how this has affected nurses capacity to respond to hospital reform, *Nursing Inquiry*, 7(2), 120–35.

Delanty, G. (2000) *Citizenship in a Global Age: Society, Culture, Politics*. Buckingham: Open University Press.

Dent, M. (1995) Doctors, Peer Review and Quality Assurance, in T. Johnson, G. Larkin and M. Saks (eds), *Health Professions and the State in Europe*. London: Routledge, pp. 86–102.

Department of Health (1989) *Caring for People: community care in the next decade and beyond*. London: HMSO.

Department of Health (1992) *The Health of the Nation: a strategy for health in England*. London: HMSO.

Department of Health (1992a) *The Health of the Nation: a strategy for health in England*. London: HMSO.

Department of Health (1992b) *The Patient's Charter*. London:HMSO.

Department of Health (1997) *The New NHS: modern, dependable*. London: The Stationery Office.

Department of Health (1999) *Saving Lives: Our Healthier Nation*. London: The Stationery Office.

Department of Health (2000) *Modernising Regulation in the Health Professions*. London: The Stationery Office.

Department of Health (2000) *The NHS Guide*. London: The Stationery Office.

Department of Health (2000) *The NHS Plan: a plan for investment, a plan for reform*. London: The Stationery Office.

Department of Health (2001) *Establishing the New Nursing and Midwifery Council*. London: The Stationery Office.

Department of Health (2001) General Social Care Council. >http://www.doh.gov.uk/gscc/info.html<

Dickenson, D. (1999) Can medical criteria settle priority-setting debates? *Health Care Analysis*, 7(2), 131–7.

Dixon, J., Harrison, A. and New, B. (1997) Is the NHS underfunded?, *British Medical Journal*, **314**, 58–61.

Dombeck, M-T. (1997) Professional personhood: training, territoriality and tolerance, *Journal of Interprofessional Care*, **11**(1), 9–21.

Donnelly, L. (1999) All hands on deck, *Health Service Journal*, **109**(5638), 9–10.

Doyal, L. (2001) Clinical ethics committees and the formulation of health care policy, *Journal of Medical Ethics*, **27** (Suppl. 1), 44–9.

Doyal, L. and Gough, I. (1991) *A Theory of Human Need*. London: Macmillan – now Palgrave Macmillan.

Duncan, P. (1999) Making sense of mortality: a qualitative study of practitioners writing about ethical problems of health promotion, *Health Education Journal*, **58**(3), 249–58.

Dunleavy, P. and O'Leary, B. (1987) *Theories of the State: The Politics of Liberal Democracy.* Basingstoke: Macmillan – now Palgrave Macmillan.

Edelstein, L. (1989) The Hippocratic Oath: text, translation and interpretation, in R.M. Veatch (ed.), *Cross Cultural Perspectives in Medical Ethics.* Boston: Jones & Bartlett.

Edwards, J. (1996) Parenting Skills: views of community health and social services providers about the needs of their clients, *Journal of Social Policy,* **24**(2), 237–59.

Edwards, S. (1996) *Nursing Ethics: a principle-based approach.* Basingstoke: Macmillan – now Palgrave Macmillan.

Edwards, S. (2001) Benner and Wrubel on caring in Nursing, *Journal of Advanced Nursing,* **33**(2), 167–71.

Ehrenreich, B. and English, D. (1973) *Witches, Midwives and Nurses: a history of women healers.* London: Writers and Readers Publishing Co-operative.

Ellis, K., Davis, A. and Rummery, K. (1999) Needs assessment, street-level bureaucracy and the new community care, *Social Policy and Administration,* **33**(3), 262–80.

Ellis, R. and Whittington, D. (1993) *Quality Assurance in Health Care: a handbook.* London: Edward Arnold.

Emanuel, E. (1991) *The Ends of Human Life.* Cambridge, MA: Harvard University Press.

Ewles, L. and Simnett, I. (1995) *Promoting Health: A Practical Guide.* London: Scutari.

Fagermoen, M. (1997) Professional Identity: values embedded in meaningful nursing practice, *Journal of Advanced Nursing,* **25**(3), 434–41.

Faulks, K. (1998) *Citizenship in Modern Britain.* Edinburgh: Edinburgh University Press.

Fedoruk, M. and Pincombe, J. (2000) The nurse executive: challenges for the 21st century, *Journal of Nursing Management,* **8**(1), 13–20.

Ferriman, A. (1999) UK government finalises restrictions on Viagra prescribing, *British Medical Journal,* **318**, 1305.

Finch, J. (1989) *Family Obligations and Social Change.* Cambridge: Polity Press.

Finch, J. and Mason, J. (1993) *Negotiating Family Responsibilities.* New York: Chapman & Hall.

Foster, P. (1996) Inequalities and Health: What health systems can and cannot do, *Journal of Health Service Research and Policy,* **1**(3), 179–82.

Fox, N. (1999) *Beyond Health: Postmodernism and Embodiment.* London: Free Association Books.

Francome, C. and Marks, D. (1996) *Improving the Health of the Nation.* London: Middlesex University Press.

Freidson, E. (1970) *Profession of Medicine.* New York: Dodds Mead.

Freire, P. (1972) *Pedagogy of the Oppressed.* Harmondsworth: Penguin.

French, P. (1979) The corporation as a moral person, *American Philosophical Quarterly,* **16**(3), 297–317.

French, P. (1984) *Collective and Corporate Responsibility.* New York: Columbia University Press.

Fuchs, L. (1990) *The American Kalaedoscope: Race, Ethnicity and the Civic Culture.* Hanover: Weslyan University Press.

Gadamer, H. (1996) *The Enigma of Health.* Cambridge: Polity Press.

General Medical Council (2002) The Duties of a Doctor, in *Guidance on Good Practice* >http://www.gmc-uk.org<

General Social Care Council (2002) *Draft Code of Practice for Social Care Workers* >http://www.doh.gov.uk/gscc/info.html<

Gibb, M. and Pryde, K. (2001) Debate: are our values safe? *Community Care,* 27 September, 25.

Giddens, A (1991) *Modernity and Self-Identity.* Cambridge: Polity Press.

Giddens, A. (1992) *The Transformation of Intimacy: sexuality, love and eroticism in modern societies.* Cambridge: Polity Press.

Giddens, A. (1998) *The Third Way: The renewal of social democracy.* Cambridge: Polity Press.

Gilligan, C. (1982) *In a Different Voice: psychological theory and women's development.* Cambridge MA: Harvard University Press.

Gitlin, T. (1993) The rise of 'identity politics', *Dissent,* **40,** 172–7.

Grantham, D. (1998) *Recent America: the United States since 1945.* Wheeling, IL: Harlan Davidson.

Gray, J. (1995) *Liberalism.* Buckingham: Open University Press.

Green, D. (1999) Solidarity Without Public Sector Monopoly: User empowerment through mutuality, in T. Ling (ed.), *Reforming Health Care by Consent.* Abingdon: Radcliffe, pp. 53–64.

Gulland, A. (2001) Doctor wins seat in fight to save hospital, *British Medical Journal,* **322,** 1443.

Gwyn, R. (1999) 'Killer bugs', 'silly buggers' and 'politically correct pals': competing discourse in health scare reporting, *Health,* **3**(3), 335–45.

Habermas, H.J. (1976) *Legitimation Crisis.* London: Heinemann.

Habermas, H.J. (1991) *Communication and the Evolution of Society* Cambridge: Polity Press.

Hallam, J. (1998) From angels to handmaidens: changing constructions of nursing's public image in post-war Britain, *Nursing Inquiry,* **5**(1), 32–42.

Ham, C. (1998) The Background, in C. Ham (ed.), *Health Care Reform: Learning From International Experience.* Buckingham: Open University Press.

Ham, C. (1999) *Health Policy in Britain.* Basingstoke: Macmillan – now Palgrave Macmillan.

Ham, C. and McIver, S. (2000) *Contested Decisions: Priority-Setting in the NHS.* London: King's Fund.

Harding, L. (1994) Parental responsibility, a dominant theme in British child and family policy for the 1990s, *International Journal of Sociology and Social Policy,* **14**(1–2), 84–108.

Harrison, A. (2000) Is there any point in spending money on reducing waiting lists? *Journal of Health Service Research and Policy,* **5**(1), 64.

Held, D. (1995) *Democracy and the Global Order: From the modern state to cosmopolitan governance.* Cambridge: Polity Press.

Helman, C. (1994) *Culture, Health and Illness: An Introduction for Health Professionals,* 3rd edn. Oxford: Butterworth-Heinemann.

Henderson, L., Kitzinger, J. and Green, J. (2000) Representing infant feeding: content analysis of British medical portrayals of bottle feeding and breast feeding, *British Medical Journal,*321, 1196–8.

Henry, C. (1995) Professional Ethics and organisational change, in K. Soothill, L. Mackay and C. Webb (eds), *Interprofessional Relations in Health Care.* London: Arnold, pp. 253–66.

Hewison, A. (2001) Values in the National Health Service: implications for nurse managers, *Journal of Nursing Management*, **9**(5), 253–8.

Hewitt, R. (1986) *White Talk Black Talk: inter-racial friendship and communication among adolescents.* Cambridge: Cambridge University Press.

Heyman, B. (1998) Introduction, in B. Heyman (ed.), *Risk, Health and Health Care: a qualitative approach.* London: Arnold, pp. 1–23.

Hiscock, J. and Pearson, M. (1999) Looking inwards, looking outwards: dismantling the Berlin wall between health and social services, *Social Policy and Administration*, **33**(2), 150–63.

Hogg, C. and Williamson, C. (2001) Whose Interests do Lay People Represent? Towards an understanding of the role of lay people as members of committees, *Health Expectations*, **4**(1), 2–9.

Hope, T., Hicks, N., Reynolds, D., Crisp, R. and Griffiths, S. (1998) Rationing and the Health Authority, *British Medical Journal*, **317**, 1067–9.

Hope, T., Sprigings, D. and Crisp, R. (1993) 'Not clinically indicated': patients interests or resource allocation? *British Medical Journal*, **306**, 379–81.

Hudson, B. (2000) Social services and primary care groups: a window of collaborative opportunity? *Health and Social Care in the Community*, **8**(4), 242–50.

Hugman, R. and Smith, D. (1995) Ethical issues in social work: an overview, in R. Hugman & D. Smith (eds), *Ethical Issues in Social Work.* London: Routledge.

Hunter, D. (1997) *Desperately Seeking Solutions.* London: Addison-Wesley Longman.

Hurley, J., Birch, S., Stoddart, G. and Torrance, G. (1997) Medical Necessity, Benefit and Resource Allocation in Health Care, *Journal of Health Service Research and Policy*, **2**(4), 223–8.

Hutton, W. (2000) *New Life for Health: the commission in the NHS.* London: Vintage.

Iliffe, S. (2000) Nursing and the future of primary care, *British Medical Journal*, **320**, 1020–21.

Illich, I. (1995) *Limits to Medicine: Medical nemesis – the expropriation of health.* London: Marion Boyars.

Jannsens, M. and Brett, J. (1997) Meaningful Participation in Transnational Teams, *European Journal of Work and Organisational Psychology*, **6**(2), 153–68.

Johnson, D. and Johnson, F. (1987) *Joining Together: group theory and group skills*, 3rd edn. London: Prentice-Hall.

Johnson, M. and Cullen, L. (2000) Solidarity Put to the Test: Health and social care in the UK, *International Journal of Social Welfare*, 9(4), 228–37.

Johnson, T. (1996) Governmentality and the institutionalisation of expertise, in T. Johnson, G. Larkin and M. Saks (eds), *Health Professions and the State in Europe*. London: Routledge, pp. 7–24.

Jones, H. (1997) *Health and Society in 20th century Britain*. London: Longman.

Jordan, B. (1990) *Social Work in an Unjust Society*. Hemel Hempstead: Harvester Wheatsheaf.

Kingham, M. (1998) Risk imagery and the AIDS epidemic, in B. Heyman (ed.), *Risk, Health and Health care: a Qualitative approach*. London: Arnold, pp. 119–38.

Klein, R. (1995) *The New Politics of the National Health Service*. 3rd edn. London: Longman.

Klein, R., Day, P. and Redmayne, S. (1996) *Managing Scarcity: Priority setting and rationing in the national health service*, Buckingham: Open University Press.

Knowles, M. (1990) *The Adult Learner: a neglected species*, 4th edn. Houston: Gulf Publishing.

Kuhse, H. (1997) *Caring: Nurses, Women and Ethics*. Oxford: Blackwell.

Kuhse, H., Singer, P., Rickard, J., Cannold, L. and van Dyck, J. (1997) Partial and impartial ethical reasoning in health care professionals, *Journal of Medical Ethics*, **23**(4), 226–32.

Kymlicka, W. (2000) Nation-building and minority rights: comparing west and east, *Journal of Ethnic and Migration Studies*, **26**(2), 173–82.

Langan, M. (1993) The rise and fall of social work, in J. Clarke (ed.), *A Crisis in Care? Challenges to social work*. London:Sage, pp. 47–66.

Larkin, G. (1983) *Occupational Monopoly and Modern Medicine*. London: Tavistock.

Larmore, C. (1994) Pluralism and reasonable disagreement, in E. Paul, F. Miller and J. Paul (eds), *Cultural Pluralism and Moral Knowledge*. New York: Cambridge University Press.

Laurent, C. (2000) A nursing theory for nursing leadership, *Journal of Nursing Management*, **8**(2), 83–7.

Leat, D. and Perkins, E. (1998) Juggling and Dealing: the creative work of care package purchasing, *Social Policy and Administration*, **32**(2), 166–81.

Lee, M. (1993) *Consumer Culture Reborn*. London: Routledge.

Light, D. (2001) Management competition, governmentality and institutional response in the United Kingdom, *Social Science and Medicine*, **52**(8), 1167–81.

Lin, N. (1973) *The Study of Human Communication*. Indianapolis: Bobbs-Merrill.

Lipsky, M. (1980) *Street-Level Bureaucracy*. New York: Russell Sage.

Lister, R. (1998) From equality to inclusion: new labour and the welfare state, *Critical Social Policy*, **18**(2), 215–25.

Loughlin, M. (1996) *Legality and Locality: the role of law in central-local government relations.* Oxford: Clarendon.

Lukes, S. (1974) *Power: a Radical View.* London: Macmillan – now Palgrave Macmillan.

Lund, B. (1999) Ask not what your community can do for you: obligations, new labour and welfare reform, *Critical Social Policy,* 19(4), 447–62.

Lupton, D. (1995) *The Imperative of Health: public health and the regulated body.* London: Sage.

MacKay, L. (1993) *Conflicts in Care: Medicine and nursing.* London: Chapman and Hall.

March, J. (1999) *The Pursuit of Organisational Intelligence.* Malden MA: Blackwell.

Marriner-Tomey, A. (1989) *Nursing Theorists and Their Work,* 2nd edn. St Louis: Mosby.

Marshall, T.H. (1950) *Citizenship, Social Class and Other Essays,* Cambridge: Cambridge University Press.

Martensen, R. (2001) The history of bioethics: an essay review, *Journal of the History of Medicine and Allied Sciences,* 56(2), 168–75.

Mast, M. and van Atta, M. (1986) Applying adult learning principles in instructional module design, *Nurse Educator,* 11(1), 35–9.

May, W. (1975) Code, covenant, contract or philanthropy, *Hastings Center Reports,* 5(1), 29–38.

Mays, N. (2000) Legitimate Decision-making: the Achilles heel of solidaristic health care, *Journal of Health Service Research and Policy,* 5(2), 122–6.

McBean, S. (1997) Health and Health Promotion: Consensus and Conflict, in A. Perry (ed.), *Nursing: A Knowledge Base for Practice.* London: Arnold.

McConaghy, J. and Cottone, R. (1998) The systemic view of violence: an ethical perspective, *Family Process,* 37(1), 51–64.

Meads, G. and Ashcroft, J. (2000) *Relationships in the NHS: bridging the gap.* London: RSM Press.

Meleis, A. (1997) *Theoretical Nursing: developments and progress,* 3rd edn. Philadelphia: Lippincott.

Mill, J.S. (1962) Utilitarianism, in M. Warnock (ed.), *Utilitarianism.* London: Collins.

Miller, D. (1976) *Social Justice.* Oxford: Clarendon Press.

Moss, H. and Siegler, M. (1991) Should alcoholics compete equally for liver transplantation?, *Journal of the American Medical Association,* 265(10), 1295–8.

Mouffe, C. (1993) *The Return of the Political.* London: Verso.

Navarro, V. (1994) *The Politics of Health Policy.* Cambridge MA: Blackwell.

Neighbour, R. (1997) *The Inner Consultation: how to develop an effective and intuitive consulting style.* Plymouth: Petroc Press.

Nelson, S. (2001) From salvation to civics: service to the sick in nursing discourse, *Social Science & Medicine,* 53(9), 1217–25.

Nettleton, S. (1995) *Sociology of Health and Illness.* Cambridge: Polity Press.

Nicoll, L. (1997) *Perspectives on Nursing Theory*, 3rd edn. Philadelphia: Lippincott.

Noddings, N. (1986) *Caring: A feminine approach to ethics and moral education*. Berkeley CA: University of California Press.

Nortvedt, P. (2001) Needs, closeness and responsibilities: an inquiry into some rival moral considerations in nursing care, *Nursing Philosophy*, **2**(2), 112–21.

Nursing and Midwifery Council (NMC) (2002) *Code of Professional Conduct*. London: NMC.

O'Brien, M. (1995) Health and Lifestyle: A critical mess? Notes on the dedifferentiation of health, in R. Bunton, S. Nettleton and R. Burrows (eds), *The Sociology of Health Promotion: Critical Analyses of Consumption, Lifestyle and Risk*, London: Routledge, pp. 191–205.

O'Brien, M. and Penna, S. (1998) *Theorising Welfare: enlightenment and modern society*. London: Sage.

Oliver, A. (2001) Increasing National Health Service Funding: Implications for welfare and justice, *Journal of Public Health Medicine*, **23**(1), 7–10.

Ovretveit, J. (1993) *Co-ordinating Community Care: Multidisciplinary teams and care management*. Buckingham: Open University Press.

Pahl, R. (1995) Friendly Society, *New Statesman and Society*, 10 March, 20–22.

Parekh, B. (1998) Integrating Minorities, in T. Blackstone, B. Parekh and P. Sanders, (eds), *Race Relations in Britain*. London: Routledge.

Parsons, T. (1939) The professions and the social structure, *Social Forces*, **17**(8), 457–67.

Parsons, T. (1972) Definitions of health and illness in the light of American values and social structure, in E. Jaco and E. Gartley (eds), *Patients, Physicians and Illness: a sourcebook in behavioural science and health*. London: Collier-Macmillan, pp. 97–117

Paton, H.J. (1978) *The Moral Law: Kant's 'Groundwork of the Metaphysic of Morals'*. London: Hutchinson.

Pattison, S. (2001) Are nursing codes of practice ethical? *Nursing Ethics*, **8**(1), 5–18.

Pellegrino, E. (1989) Toward an expanded medical ethics: the Hippocratic Oath revisited, in R.M. Veatch. (ed.), *Cross Cultural Perspectives in Medical Ethics*. Boston: Jones & Bartlett.

Persaud, R. (1995) Smokers rights to health care, *Journal of Medical Ethics*, **21**(5), 281–7.

Petersen, A. (2001) Biofantasies: genetics and medicine in the print news media, *Social Science & Medicine*, **52**(8), 1255–68.

Pickard, S. and Sheaff, R. (1999) Primary Care Groups and NHS Rationing: Implications of the Child B Case, *Health Care Analysis*, **7**(1), 37–56.

Pilgrim, D. (1995) Explaining abuse and inadequate care, in G. Hunt (ed.), *Whistleblowing in the Health Service*. London: Arnold, pp. 77–88.

Plant, R. (1992) Citizenship, rights and welfare, in A. Coote (ed.), The Welfare of Citizens. London: Institute of Public Policy Research, pp. 15–30.

Powell, M. (2000) Analysing the 'new' British National Health Service, *International Journal of Health Planning and Management*, **15**(2), 89–101.

Pritchard, P. (1995) Learning to work effectively in teams, in P.Owens, J. Carrier, and J. Horder (eds), *Interprofessional Issues in Community and Primary Health Care*. Basingstoke: Macmillan – now Palgrave Macmillan, pp. 205–32.

Rafferty, M. (1992) Nursing Policy and the Nationalisation of Nursing, in J. Robinson, A. Gray and R. Elkan (eds), *Policy Issues in Nursing*. Buckingham: Open University Press.

Rains, J. and Barton-Kriese, P. (2001) Developing political competence: a comparative study across disciplines, *Public Health Nursing*, **18**(4), 219–24.

Rawls, J. (1971) *A Theory of Justice*. New York: Oxford University Press.

Rawls, J. (1993) *Political Liberalism*. New York: Columbia University Press.

Richardson, R. and Waddington, C. (1996) Allocating resources: community involvement is not easy, *International Journal of Health Planning and Management*, **11**(4), 307–15.

Robertson, D. (1996) Ethical theory, ethnography and differences between doctors and nurses approaches to patient care, *Journal of Medical Ethics*, **22**(5), 292–9.

Rorty, R. (1994) *Contingency, Irony and Solidarity*. Cambridge: Cambridge University Press.

Ryan, A. (1991) Merit Goods and Benefits in Kind: Paternalism and liberalism in action, in T. Wilson and D. Wilson (eds), *The State and Social Welfare*. London: Longman, pp. 89–104.

Schwarzmantel, J. (1994) *The State in Contemporary Society*. London: Harvester Wheatsheaf.

Seebohm Report (1968) *Report of the Committee on Local Authority and Allied Personal Social Services*. London: HMSO.

Seedhouse, D. (1986) *Health: The Foundations for Achievement*. London: Wiley.

Seedhouse, D. (1991) *Liberating Medicine*. Chichester: Wiley.

Seedhouse, D. (1997) *Health Promotion: Philosophy, prejudice and practice*. Chichester: Wiley.

Seedhouse, D. (2000) *Practical Nursing Philosophy: the universal ethical code*. New York: Wiley.

Seligman, A. (1993) The Fragile Ethical Vision of Civil Society, in B. Turner (ed.), Citizenship and Social Theory. London: Sage.

Senge, P. (1994) *The Fifth Discipline: the art and practice of the learning organisation*. New York: Currency Doubleday.

Sheaff, R. (1999) The Development of English Primary Care Group Governance: a scenario analysis, *International Journal of Health Planning and Management*, **14**(4), 257–68.

Slowther, A., Bunch, C., Woolnough, B. and Hope, T. (2001) Clinical ethics support services in the UK: an investigation of the current provision of ethics support to health professionals in the UK, *Journal of Medical Ethics*, **27** (Suppl. 1), 2–18.

Smith, G. (1979) *Social Work and The Sociology of Organisations*. London: Routledge & Kegan Paul.

Smith, L. and Morrissey, J. (1994) Ethical dilemmas for General Practitioners under the new UK contract, *Journal of Medical Ethics*, **20**(3), 175–80.

Smith, P., Masterson, A. and Lloyd Smith, S. (1999) Health promotion versus disease and care: failure to establish 'blissful clarity' in British nurse education and practice, *Social Science and Medicine*, **48**(2), 227–40.

Sorrell, T. (2001) Citizen-patient/citizen-doctor, *Health Care Analysis*, **9**(1), 25–39.

Stalker, K., Baron, S., Riddell, S. and Wilkinson, H. (1999) Models of disability: the relationship between theory and practice in non-statutory organisations, *Critical Social Policy*, **19**(1), 5–29.

Stevenson, C. and Beech, I. (2001) Paradigms lost, paradigms regained:-defending nursing against a single reading of postmodernism, *Nursing Philosophy*, **2**(2), 143–50.

Svensson, J. (1996) The interplay between doctors and nurses, *Sociology of Health and Illness*, **18**(3), 379–98.

Tawney, R.H. (1990) *Religion and the Rise of Capitalism*. London: Penguin.

The Stationery Office (1998) *The Public Interest Disclosure Act*. London: The Stationery Office.

Tonnies, F. (1955) *Community and Association*. London: Routledge & Kegan Paul.

Toon, P. (1994) Justice for Gatekeepers, *Lancet*, **343**, 585–7.

Tschudin, V. and Hunt, G. (1997) Editorial, *Nursing Ethics*, **4**(4), 265–7.

Underwood, M. and Bailey, J. (1993) Coronary bypass surgery should not be offered to smokers, *British Medical Journal*, **306**, 1047–50.

United Kingdom Central Council (UKCC) for Nursing, Midwifery and Health Visiting (1992) *Code of Professional Conduct for the Nurse, Midwife and Health Visitor*, 3rd edn. London: UKCC.

United Nations (1948) *Universal Declaration of Human Rights*. Geneva: UN.

van Dyne, L. and Saavedra, R. (1996) A naturalistic minority influence experiment: effects on divergent thinking, conflict and originality in work-groups, *British Journal of Social Psychology*, **35**(1), 151–67.

van Hooft, S. (1999) Acting from the virtue of caring in nursing, *Nursing Ethics*, **6**(3), 189–201.

Velasquez, M. (1983) Why corporations are not morally responsible for what they do, *Business and Professional Ethics Journal*, **2**, 1–18.

Walby, S. and Greenwell, J. (with Mackay, L. and Soothill, K.) (1994) *Medicine and Nursing: professions in a changing Health Service*. London: Sage.

Weber, M. (1923) *Economic History.* London: Allen & Unwin.

Weber, M. (1978) *Economy and Society.* Berkeley, CA: University of California Press.

Wells, J. (1999) The growth of managerialism and its impact on Nursing and the NHS, in I. Norman and S. Cowley (eds), *The Changing Nature of Nursing in a Managerial Age.* Oxford: Blackwell, pp. 57–81.

Welsh, T. and Pringle, M. (2001) Social capital: trusts need to recreate trust, *British Medical Journal,* **323**, 177–8.

West, M. (1997) Collaboration improves the quality of care. Conference Paper, Journal of Interprofessional Care Conference 'All Together Better Health', London, 18 July.

White, B. (1994) *Competence to Consent.* Washington: Georgetown University Press.

White, R. (1985) *The Effects of the NHS on the Nursing Profession.* London: King's Fund.

Wicks, D. (1998) *Nurses and Doctors at Work.* Buckingham: Open University Press.

Williams, A. (1985) Economics of coronary artery bypass grafting, *British Medical Journal,* **291**, 326–9.

Williams, A. (2000) *Nursing, Medicine and Primary Care.* Buckingham: Open University Press.

Wilmot, S. (1997) *The Ethics of Community Care.* London: Cassell.

Wilmot, S. (1998) Nursing by agreement: a contractarian perspective on nursing ethics, *Advanced Practice Nursing Quarterly,* **4**(2), 1–7.

Wilmot, S. (2000) Corporate moral responsibility in health care, *Medicine, Health Care and Philosophy,* **3**(2), 139–46.

Wilson, D. and Game, C. (1998) *Local Government in the United Kingdom.* Basingstoke: Macmillan – now Palgrave Macmillan.

World Health Organization (1946) *Constitution.* Geneva: WHO.

World Medical Association (1989) Declaration of Geneva, in R.M. Veatch (ed.), *Cross Cultural Perspectives in Medical Ethics.* Boston: Jones & Bartlett.

Index